Ritalin-Free
Kids

ALSO BY THE AUTHORS

The Patient's Guide to
Homeopathic Medicine
and
Homeopathic Self-Care

———⟋⊗⟍———

Ritalin-Free Kids

Safe and Effective Homeopathic Medicine for ADD and Other Behavioral and Learning Problems

Judyth Reichenberg-Ullman, N.D., M.S.W.

Robert Ullman, N.D.

PRIMA HEALTH
A Division of Prima Publishing

This book is intended for educational purposes only. It is not intended to diagnose, treat, give medical advice for a specific condition, or in any way to replace the services of a qualified medical practitioner. When making general references to our patients we alternate "he" and "she" for the purpose of equality of gender reference.

The cases in this book are true stories from our clinical practice. We have tried as much as possible to use the words of the patients and to tell their stories as they were told to us. We have changed the names to protect confidentiality.

Library of Congress Cataloging-in-Publication Data

Reichenberg-Ullman, Judyth.
    Ritalin-free kids : safe and effective homeopathic medicine for ADD and other behavioral and learning problems / by Judyth Reichenberg-Ullman and Robert Ullman.
        p.   cm.
    Includes index.
    ISBN 0-7615-0719-1
    1. Attention-deficit hyperactivity disorder—Homeopathic treatment.
    2. Attention-deficit hyperactivity disorder—Chemotherapy—Complications.
    3. Methylphenidate hydrochloride—Side effects.   I. Reichenberg-Ullman, Judyth.   II. Title.
    RX531.A77U45   1996
    616.85'8906—dc20   96-28572
                                                                                          CIP

        99 00 HH 10 9
Printed in the United States of America

How to Order:
Single copies may be ordered from Prima Publishing, P.O. Box 1260BK, Rocklin, CA 95677; telephone (916) 632-4400. Quantity discounts are also available. On your letterhead, include information concerning the intended use of the books and the number of books you wish to purchase.

Visit us online at http:\\www.primahealth.com

*We dedicate this book to our parents,
who raised us with love, support, and
guidance, and particularly to Judyth's mother,
eighty-six-year-old Essie Reichenberg, our
biggest fan and only living parent.*

*We also dedicate this book to the many children
whom we have enjoyed seeing as patients and
whose stories appear in this book, and to their
parents for having the open-mindedness and
trust to seek out homeopathy.*

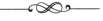

Contents

PART TWO
Homeopathy: A Whole Person Approach

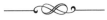

Foreword

In some schools 30 percent of the children are on Ritalin. Does this epidemic of attention deficit hyperactive disorder reflect something new? Are we just diagnosing better? Are the latent weaknesses of the human nervous system becoming overwhelmed by the pace and complexity of life in the information age? No one has enough time. We are flooded with sound and video bytes. There is more to do than anyone has time for. Kids don't have time or space to be kids. The expectations are enormous. Each of us can experience how our nervous systems are overflowing with the stress this environment creates. While there are similarities, each of us has our own unique way of coping and adapting.

People with ADHD manifest their distress differently depending on their unique constitutions. Many are overstimulated, distracted, and restless. Others become hypervigilant, withdrawn, and compulsive. Others act out, become disruptive or aggressive. All have trouble with self-esteem in their struggle to function. All these various presentations might be labeled as ADHD. Despite the diversity, the conventional approach boils the problem down into a single diagnosis, which is typically treated by a single class of drugs. As long as medications are continued, the symptoms are somewhat controlled, much to the relief of the child or adult, teachers, and parents. Few patients ever outgrow their need for drug therapy. Many stop because of the side effects, limited effectiveness, or to try something different. Before you give your child stimulants, read this book. This book describes another approach—one that respects and takes advantage of the diversity of people with symptoms of ADHD: an approach that stimulates the unique adaptive mechanisms each person carries within. Homeopathy is a system of medicine that is highly individualized and can help people move toward more optimal health. The case examples in this book demonstrate that, when used alone or as a complement to conventional therapies, homeopathic medicines can improve the function of people with ADHD to the point where conventional medicines are often no longer necessary.

The authors describe their experience with more than 400 ADHD patients whom they have treated. The words of the patients tell the story. Positive evidence is accumulating from clinical and laboratory studies to support the claims of homeopathy. Much more rigorous research is needed into the homeopathic approach before it gains wider acceptance. The clinical experience described in this book will undoubtedly catch the eye of those who have the resources to devote to scientific inquiry. The goal of medical research is to bring safe and effective therapies to the public. The evidence provided by these two pioneering practitioners will undoubtedly stimulate the dialogue between conventional and complementary health care providers, to the benefit of both.

For those who need support in their struggle with ADHD and can't wait for the years of research, they can be assured from two hundred years experience using homeopathic medicines that they are safe. Make your own judgments about effectiveness based on the patients' stories presented. Your conventional doctor may be skeptical if you choose to use homeopathy. Don't let that stop you, or stop you from telling him or her. Your doctor will then have the chance to grow with you. But take the advice of the authors and seek assistance from well-trained homeopathic providers who are willing to work with you and your doctors. Then everyone stands to learn and benefit.

Edward H. Chapman, M.D., Dht
President, American Institute of Homeopathy
Clinical Instructor, Harvard University
    School of Medicine
Investigator in the NIH funded research—The Homeopathic Treatment of Mild Traumatic Brain Injury

Acknowledgments

Special thanks to Miranda Castro, FsHom, for her encouragement and support and for providing excellent feedback on the first draft of our manuscript. We particularly thank Ted Chapman for writing the foreword. Thanks to Leslie Howle for her loving friendship and for her wisdom about children. We thank Shane McCamey for heartily encouraging us to write this book and for his unshakable confidence that this book will bring many more parents and children to homeopathy. We thank Jennifer Jacobs, M.D., M.P.H., Richard Solomon, M.D., and Dana Ullman, M.P.H. for generously offering their time to review our book. We are especially grateful to Rajan Sankaran, Jayesh Shah, Nandita Shah, Sujit Chatterjee, Divya Chhabra, and Sunil Anand for inspiring us in their brilliant method of classical homeopathy.

Introduction

Attention deficit hyperactivity disorder (ADD or ADHD) is being diagnosed in epidemic proportions. According to a recent Public Broadcasting System documentary, at least two million children in the United States are currently taking stimulant medications (including Ritalin, Dexedrine, and Cylert) for ADD. That is more than one in every thirty children ages five to eighteen. In 1988 half a million children were being prescribed stimulants for ADD. The number has quadrupled in only eight years and is doubling every two years. Physicians in this country prescribe five times the quantity of stimulants for children as the rest of the countries of the world combined. These are regulated by the Drug Enforcement Agency (DEA).[1] A recent report by the United Nations revealed that 3 to 5 percent of all U.S. schoolchildren are taking Ritalin.[2] In 1990, the number of children diagnosed with ADD was 750,000. Today the figure is approaching four million. Ciba-Geigy, the company that manufactures Ritalin, attributes the surge in ADD to "heightened public

---

[1]The Merrow Report: *ADD-A Dubious Diagnosis.* Public Broadcasting System. October 20, 1994.
[2] "Misuse of Ritalin by Schoolchildren Prompts Warning," *Seattle Times,* March 27, 1996.

awareness." Much of that awareness, however, appears to have been created by Ciba-Geigy itself, a large contributor to ADD support groups throughout the United States, which often recommends medication to parents.[3]

Production of Ritalin has increased by nearly 500 percent in the last five years according to the DEA.[4] Dr. James Swanson, director of the Child Development Center at the University of California, Irvine, states that the sudden increase in Ritalin use is cause for alarm. He estimates that one-third of these children should not be taking it.[5] Dr. Lawrence Diller, a behavioral pediatrician practicing in Walnut Creek, California, has said he was scared to see even three- or four-year-old children taking the drug.[6]

Imagine the following scenario: eight-year-old Johnny has just entered second grade. His teacher quickly notices that he is forever wriggling around in his seat and simply cannot keep his hands off of the children around him. He disrupts the class by asking questions all the time. Johnny crawls under his desk and refuses to come out. He has a terrible time paying attention to the teacher's instructions and he cannot seem to follow through on completing homework and turning in assignments. His handwriting is a disaster. Within a matter of weeks, if Johnny's teacher is patient, his parents start receiving notes from the teacher reporting his disruptive behaviors. Within two months, the teacher asks to have a conference with Johnny's parents. "Have you heard of ADD?" she asks. "Have you thought of putting your child on Ritalin?" Johnny's bewildered parents leave feeling

---

[3]"Merrow Report Questions ADD Diagnosis," *Latitudes,* 2 (1996):1.
[4]"Boom in Ritalin Sales Raises Ethical Issues," *New York Times,* May 15, 1966.
[5]Ibid.
[6]Ibid.

an array of emotions, ranging from frustration with their child, anger at the teacher for suggesting that Johnny needed drugs, and doubts about whether they have done something wrong in their parenting.

Many of these parents end up in the office of their family physician, a psychologist, or a psychiatrist seeking prescriptions for stimulants for their children. Other parents initially refuse to consider giving drugs to their children, then change their minds out of fear that they will ruin their children's opportunities to learn and mature normally. Once children like Johnny begin taking stimulants, they often need to continue the medication for five to ten years, sometimes for life.

We offer an alternative to Ritalin and other stimulant medications to those of you who have ADD or have children diagnosed with ADD. BEFORE YOU FILL THAT PRESCRIPTION FOR STIMULANTS, READ THIS BOOK! Homeopathic medicine is a safe, effective, and natural treatment for ADD and an approach that may be entirely new to you and your family (see chapter 7). If you are inspired by this book, which is our hope, please find an experienced homeopath to treat you or your child. DO NOT USE THE INFORMATION IN THIS BOOK TO SELF-PRESCRIBE FOR ADD. Homeopathic prescribing is an art as well as a science. The success and long-lasting results which you see in this book and which you may be seeking are only possible under the care of a qualified homeopathic practitioner.

We began treating children with ADD nine years ago. We were astounded at how homeopathy transformed the lives of many of these children in a very positive way. Jimmy was one of the first children with ADD whom we treated homeopathically. Here is his story:

Jimmy was a nine-year-old child diagnosed with ADD. His parents, both in their fifties, had been in and out of alcoholism treatment programs. Jimmy and his younger sister had been shuffled from one foster home to another. Both children had been routinely beaten and subjected to profound neglect. Jimmy was afraid to go into the bathroom because that was where his mother used to beat him. When Jimmy arrived at the home of the foster mother who brought him to see us, he was filthy. He had not had a haircut for a year. His shoes were three and a half sizes too small.

Jimmy's behavior was extreme. He was active and busy all the time. He had been placed in special education classes due to his disruptive classroom behavior. He jumped up and down constantly, pestered the other children, and drove his teacher so crazy that she insisted that Jimmy's foster mother come to school and sit with him in class all day, or he could not attend.

Jimmy hummed, twiddled, sang, and talked incessantly. He shook rattles, squeezed horns, and grabbed anything he could find to keep himself busy. Jimmy was always moving some part of his body. His hands fidgeted and he swung his legs restlessly. At bedtime, he jumped on and off the bed and talked to his foster sister even after she had fallen asleep. When he finally fell asleep, he tossed and turned all night.

Jimmy was extremely impatient. If taken out in public, he wandered away. Despite his uncontrollable restlessness, Jimmy was kind, considerate, and would be the first to give away his candy bar if another child did not have one.

We prescribed for Jimmy the homeopathic medicine *Veratrum album* (White hellebore). Within two days after the medication, his hyperactivity had improved dramatically. Jimmy's teacher called his foster mother to ask what she had done with him. She could take him shopping now and he no longer wandered off. He stopped humming and talking all the time and no longer chattered to his sister after she was asleep. We were able to follow Jimmy's progress for two more years, and he continued to do very well.

Because of the impressive results in Jimmy's case and several others, we began to use homeopathy with many children with ADD and other behavioral and learning problems. As we began to write articles about our successful cases, parents called us from all over the United States asking us to treat their children. We have treated nearly 400 children diagnosed with ADD, as well as a number of adults. We include many cases in our book so that you can see for yourself how effective homeopathy is with these children. We estimate our success rate to be 70 percent when the patients continue with homeopathic treatment for at least one year. People with ADD are some of our favorite patients. They can be lively, engaging, bright, entertaining, and witty. However, their extreme behaviors and tendencies often get them into lots of trouble. Treating these patients has become an extremely rewarding aspect of our practice. If either or both parents also have ADD, the family will benefit the most if each family member is treated.

This book may be your first exposure to homeopathic medicine. As you will see, prescribing homeopathic medicines for ADD is a complex but highly effective and rewarding process. If you choose to use homeopathy as a natural alternative to treat ADD, we strongly advise you to consult a qualified and experienced homeopathic practitioner.

.

PART ONE

The Conventional
View of ADD

1

---⟨∞⟩---

Drifty, Driven, and Daring
The Characteristics of ADD

Calling Planet Earth . . . Do You Read Me?

ADD is a multifaceted condition. The problems with attention and/or hyperactive and impulsive behaviors are significant enough to interfere with normal functioning in the home, school, or work environment. People with ADD do not all behave in the same way. Some are dreamy, drifty, or spaced out, without being hyperactive. They seem lost in the clouds, barely on the planet, and oblivious to most interactions. Others are on the go, bouncing off the walls, driven, and motorized. Still others have no ability to wait, interrupt constantly, have to be first, and are always seeking out something new or stimulating.

People with ADD have difficulty concentrating and paying attention in situations where they are forced to sit still, such as at school or at their desks at work. They may sit for hours reading their favorite books, playing Nintendo, watching television, or actively playing outside, but when they are required to perform tasks, do homework, write a paper, do household chores, or balance their checkbook, they may be able to concentrate

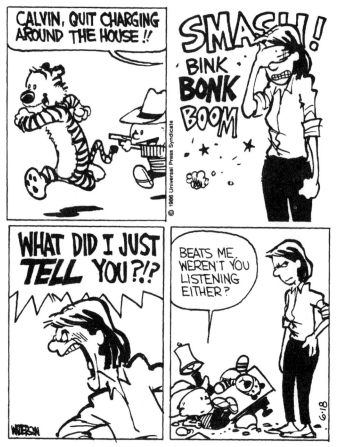

Calvin and Hobbes © (1986) Watterson. Distributed by Universal Press Syndicate. Reprinted with permission. All rights reserved.

for only a few minutes before something more interesting captures their attention.

Work tends to be hastily done, sloppy and careless, with many mistakes. It is hard for the person with ADD to listen to instructions and follow through until the task is complete. It is not that the individual does not want to finish things. He just never quite gets around to it. Things are done impulsively or not at all. Procrastination and difficulty getting started are major problems, complemented by equal difficulty with completing anything, especially on time. Many projects are started but few are finished. At certain times, though, the individual may place tremendous attention on tasks that he wants to do.

Where DID I Put That Wallet?

An ADD person's environment often looks like a tornado hit it. There are the remains of many unfinished projects and stacks of papers and objects which appear to be in utter disarray. These people tend to lose things they need like car keys, homework, important papers, checkbooks, wallets, and clothes. They insist that the objects in question are "in that pile," "around here somewhere," or "under that pizza box over there." These individuals may be careless and tend to be clumsy and break things.

In social situations, they often miss the subtle cues of facial expression, tone of voice, and body language that make up such a large part of social communication. Their attention may be so poor as to drift off and totally miss what the other person is saying, or to fade in and out, only getting enough to embarrass themselves when they try to respond to the conversation they have only barely heard. ADD causes people to have trouble making friends and more difficulty in keeping them. They forget appointments, dates, and birthdays, or show up late with a lame apology.

Wired for Sound

When hyperactivity is predominant in ADD, the person may be "wired." Excessive activity is common, especially in children, such as running back and forth through the house or climbing furniture and trees. These children often engage routinely in reckless activities that terrify their parents, such as jumping from high places, running out in traffic without looking, or just wandering off, nowhere to be seen. All children do some of these things, but for the ADD child and some adults these are constant activities, enough to drive their parents crazy with fear, worry, and exhaustion. Many parents say "She never stops going, morning, noon, and night," or "You can turn her on but you can't turn her off!" Restless squirming, fidgeting with objects, tapping fingers and feet, drumming, and pacing are all ways for the child or adult to unconsciously mark time and release nervous energy.

Act First, Think Later

Impulsivity is another major feature of the picture. Patience is not a virtue common to the individual with ADD. He can't wait for his turn, always needs to be first, and throws caution to the wind. He acts first and thinks later, usually after something is destroyed, someone is hurt, or it is too late to do the right thing. Instructions are often considered irrelevant, or are half heard. ADD people can be quite intrusive, interrupting others to blurt out a response without letting them finish their question or sentence. ADD children are often loud, verbally inappropriate, and talk too much. They cannot be quiet even when reprimanded. They push and shove to get what they want, grab things from other people, and bang into them with total abandon and disregard for injury to themselves or others.

Intelligent Underachievers

All of these characteristics, depending on the individual's age, the context, and the intensity of expression can cause significant problems. These children are often singled out in school as troublemakers, clowns, instigators, space cadets, and intelligent underachievers who never work up to their potential. Children with ADD may be quite intelligent, but cannot seem to do well in anything that requires sitting still and paying attention, or focused work in which they are not interested. They lose assignments, fail tests, and forget what they were supposed to bring to school or take home. Their grades almost never reflect their true capabilities. ADD children do much better in small groups or in one-on-one situations. They thrive on external structure, being unable to structure their own time or activities, but also chafe under too close or severe a discipline. Easily bored, these individuals constantly seek something novel in their environments to hold their interest. ADD may also be combined with learning disabilities which can negatively compound school performance.

How Many Times Do I Have to
Tell You to Clean Your Room?

At home, parents complain of having to repeat instructions over and over. Children fail to follow through consistently on the simplest chores, being so easily distracted that they completely forget whatever they were told to do moments before. They take what seems to be forever to get dressed or eat. They may simply wander off with the task undone or may try to perform three tasks at once, handling none of them well. They need extremely close supervision to get anything done. If they are punished or reprimanded, the effect does not make a dent for long. Consequences and past experience are ignored or forgotten. Tantrumming as a way to avoid uninteresting or unpleasant tasks is a common strategy for ADD children. They may want very much to pay attention or to do a good job; they just can't.

The Upside of ADD

On the positive side, many children and adults with ADD are bright and eager to please. They can be charming, spontaneous, and fun, with a fresh moment-to-moment approach to life. People often find them more entertaining than irritating when taken in small doses. Creativity runs high in people with ADD and they often have more ideas than they can actualize effectively. They may be artistically gifted and quite sensitive. These individuals look for the new and interesting things in life. They are inventive and often innovate new ways of doing things. These people take risks that others may fear to take, and make breakthroughs as a result. They may be dreamers, but their dreams can turn into a very gratifying and lucrative reality if they team up with others who are more grounded and follow through on their ideas. If provided with an interesting, flexible environment with enough structure and encouragement to follow through, people with ADD can live exciting and fulfilling lives. With effective treatment, whether conventional or alternative, their odds for enjoying and succeeding in life are greatly enhanced.

2

Life in Overdrive
Growing Up with ADD

Rug Rats on the Run

Some children give hints as early as infancy that they may have tendencies toward ADD. It is important to remember that it is much too early to diagnose positively at such a young age, and that some infants manifesting these symptoms may grow out of them in a matter of months or years. The following are symptoms that we have seen with our patients that may send up a red flag regarding future ADD.

Restlessness   Infants constantly move around, squirm, and kick. They want to be held, then put down, then picked up again. They roll about in their cribs and crawl around vigorously as soon as they can.

Poor eye contact   Their eyes dart about, unable to focus on one thing for very long. They may not attend to social cues like smiling or frowning to which their peers already respond.

Sleeplessness   ADD infants may seem never to sleep. They are hard to put to sleep and wake frequently, wanting attention. You may want some sleep but it is the last thing on your child's mind.

Frequent fussiness   Never satisfied, these children often fuss and fret, demanding constant attention and stimulation, while other children are more easily pacified and put to sleep. Whimpering or crying incessantly, they always seem to have a problem, refusing whatever is offered and generally being disagreeable.

Intensity   As a parent you may notice that infants with ADD are more demanding, labor intensive, and emotionally intense than your other children or your friends' children. You may sometimes wish they had never been born as you struggle to cope with the array of problems these special children bring with them, or you may feel equally blessed by the gifts of energy, fun, and creativity they bring as well.

Motorized Toddlers

Experts claim that we can identify 60 to 70 percent of ADD children with hyperactivity by age two to three.[1] Parents often tell us that their ADD toddlers ran before they walked! The traits they had as babies often intensified as they began to be mobile and expressive.

Toddlers on the go   Running, jumping, and climbing are all in five minutes' work for ADD toddlers. They out-

---

[1]Thomas Phelan, Ph.D., Lecture, Tukwila, WA, 1/26/96.

last the Energizer bunny and toddle faster than a speeding Hot Wheels.

Need for constant stimulation   You always have to keep these children busy or they do interesting things like crayoning all over a newly painted wall or putting the cat in the oven. They love to play, but with a new toy every two minutes. They do not have time to get bored before they are on to the next activity.

Reckless, impulsive, and accident-prone   Boys with ADD have this trait more often than girls. They seem to have no fear as they tempt death with reckless abandon, only to be rescued at the last moment by a horrified parent. One child, at three, crawled out on the roof through an open bedroom window. He nearly gave his mother a heart attack. Another boy was so accident-prone that he was rushed to the hospital twice in one day, both times for stitches in his head.

Tantrums   All children have tantrums sometimes, but ADD children can have them multiple times in a day. These are real tantrums, complete with kicking, biting, crying, screaming, flailing, and beating their heads on the floor or the nearest wall. Parents get exhausted by them, wondering when their child will ever stop and do what he or she is told.

No need for naps and hard to put to bed   The only respite for many parents is the afternoon nap and when the child is finally put to bed. Unfortunately, these children are not interested in bed. There is so much more to see, do, and experience before sleep can even be considered. It is a matter of who exhausts whom first, and it is no contest.

Demanding constant attention and being jealous
ADD children want to be noticed and do whatever they must to get the attention on which they thrive. If another child is center stage, these children can become quite jealous, and even behave maliciously to their siblings.

Hurting animals   Animals can also fall prey to the too vigorous play of ADD children, their impulsivity, lack of attention and care, and at times, cruelty or jealousy. It is wise to make sure that your child is capable of relating well to the animals in your home or neighborhood before leaving them alone together.

Pesky Preschoolers

By the time your child is three to five years old, the seeds of ADD begin to sprout even more visibly. Watch for the following behaviors to surface at home, at preschool, with the babysitter, and at family and social events.

Defiance and tantrums   All children say "no" and act out in public, but for ADD children, the behavior can be extreme and relentless. Parents become embarrassed about even taking their child to the grocery store for fear of a kicking, screaming battle over an ardently desired treat. We have even heard of parents in this kind of battle zone being accused of abusing their children, when all they were trying to do was get the child out the door without too much damage being done.

Difficulty getting along with peers   ADD children can lag behind in social skills because they do not notice the subtle cues that define interactions among children.

When other children are learning to play together and share, these children may be too annoying, bossy, or self-centered to keep friends and be included in games and parties. This can be heartbreaking for parents to witness and for the child to experience.

Violent and destructive   Venting frustration and anger leads children to express violence, by breaking their own toys or those of other children, damaging their home, their parents' treasured objects, and anything else they can get their hands on. Some children also bite, kick, hit, and scratch as they violently release their feelings.

Difficulty paying attention and following directions "He doesn't listen!" say the parents of these children. It is as if they are in another world, tuned out, or on a different wavelength. Anything can distract them from the task at hand. It can take a child half an hour to brush his teeth while he pets the dog, watches TV, bothers his sister, picks up his favorite toy, and eats a gumdrop. Every moment is full of endless opportunities for diversion. Each task has to be broken into small steps, with constant supervision, or it simply will not happen.

Complaints from preschool teachers   Children with ADD act silly, will not stop talking, fail to follow directions, will not take naps, talk back to the teacher, and get into fights with other kids when frustrated.

Mean to animals and other children   Hamsters, dogs, cats, and other small animals flee in terror from some of these kids, who have no idea why Muffy will not come near them anymore. We have heard of several unfortunate hamsters who have met their ends at the hands of an overzealous caretaker who did not understand the law of gravity. Brothers, sisters, and small friends fare little better, getting hit by a flailing fist or foot or intentionally tripped.

Mischievous ADD children can be instigators and clowns, teasing and mischievous. Their silliness is contagious. They poke, hide, play tricks, climb on the teacher's desk, crawl under the tables, steal food, and make a nuisance of themselves.

Dawdling Any parent of an ADD child knows how infuriatingly slow he or she can be. Just when you are ready to leave for an important appointment, he or she tunes out, takes forever, and is distracted by a million things. Just putting on socks can be an all-morning affair, not to mention something really complicated like eating breakfast.

Significant Problems Start at School

When your child is five to twelve years old and starts to attend school, many symptoms of ADD become even more obvious. The school environment is likely to be more rigid and demanding than what he or she has previously faced. At home the child has to cope with more responsibilities such as household chores and homework. The distinction between ADD behavior and conduct disorders may sometimes overlap.

Difficulty with reading, writing, and taking tests— poor grades Reading ability and comprehension may be difficult for the ADD child. Problems with attention and memory make it hard to learn to read and to write as well. Poor reading and writing impair learning ability. Handwriting is usually sloppy and sometimes unrecognizable. Only the child knows what is on the page and sometimes even he cannot figure it out. ADD may become obvious at school when the child's knowledge begins to be tested. Distraction, impulsivity, and restlessness are not useful skills at test time. Frustration may start early when success in school becomes harder to achieve as the material becomes more complex. Even if grades were initially good, as time goes on they often get worse and worse.

Problems following directions and completing assignments Distractibility makes it difficult for these children to follow directions for complex tasks. They will start a task, only to lose interest rapidly and begin to do something else that looks more immediately gratifying. They can forget completely what the original task was. If more than one step is required, they forget what to do next. If they are given each step at the proper time, and helped to focus, they can complete the task. Constant supervision and encouragement are necessary if anything is to be accomplished.

Forgetting to turn in homework—losing things Even if a child does his homework, it can be an ordeal just to get it to the teacher's desk. Dogs must consider homework a great delicacy, if they eat it as often as the child might lead his teacher to believe. Dogs are not the only culprits, however. Homework has ways of escaping from the ADD child's grasp that would rival Houdini's best efforts. Other important items like clothes, keys, books, report cards, lunch, and money are also lost, either temporarily or irretrievably.

Spacing out   "Earth to Johnny" is often heard as parents attempt to make contact with their child who is off exploring his or her own private galaxy of internal stimuli. Dreaminess and inattention cause the ADD child to miss out on important information, social interactions, and even danger signals in the environment. Dreaminess and inattention are hallmarks of ADD, especially for children without hyperactivity.

Annoying, repetitive, or clowning behavior   ADD children can be particularly annoying a lot of the time. They are known for relentless fidgeting and restlessness, repetitive movements, tapping, playing with any available object, doing things over and over again even when specifically told not to, and clowning around in order to attract attention, whether positive or negative.

Making inappropriate noises and gestures   Making noises and faces and other gestures which are spontaneous and out of place in polite society is typical of all children, but the ADD child can behave so impulsively, restlessly, and inappropriately causing those around him to look in vain for the "off" button.

Interrupting and blurting out   They break into any conversation with any stream of consciousness thought that enters their heads. This can be especially distracting in school when the teacher is trying to get something across to the students and does not want the class to be diverted. This leads a child with ADD to get in trouble for inappropriately interrupting, when they were just spontaneously expressing themselves without thinking of the consequences.

Missing social cues, lack of friends, isolation A big problem for ADD kids is the lack of friends. They seem slower to catch on in social situations and are often considered to be obnoxious, annoying, or too much to deal with. They are made fun of, not chosen in groups and games, and often do not get invited to parties or overnights with other children. The result is isolation and feelings of rejection that can be lifelong.

Physically awkward and clumsy Being chosen for sports and games and being good in physical education classes is dependent on focused attention and physical coordination, skills which ADD children often lack. They make up in energy what they lack in coordination, but can give up in frustration and despair.

Complaints from teachers Parents frequently receive a constant stream of notes from school about their children with ADD. These kids can cause many problems for teachers who are trying to maintain a focused classroom environment. They need closer supervision and demand much more attention than the average child. So teachers tend to complain to parents about behavior problems and learning deficits, unsuccessfully try to discipline the child, and often feel at a loss to provide a meaningful educational experience beyond simple maintenance.

Defiance Every child says "no" sometimes, but when it is the primary response to nearly every request, a pattern of clear oppositional behavior emerges. Though not typical of every ADD child, defiance is often an unconscious strategy to feel some control and power and to get more attention from significant adults.

Sneakiness, lying, and stealing   ADD children are always getting into trouble, and many lie or cover up to minimize the damage. Stealing is a tactic for getting what they do not have the skills or attention to earn.

Intentionally harmful to others—lack of conscience   Although not specifically part of the criteria for ADD, malicious behavior can be present in some of these children as an expression of their anger and frustration.

Aggravating ADDolescents

ADD during the teen years often has its greatest impact on school performance. The hyperactivity has often diminished, at least partially, and the family is usually weary of dealing with a difficult and demanding child for years. This is also the time of preparing for college or work life independent of the family, getting a driver's license, and being exposed to peer pressure regarding drugs, alcohol, and sex. Although these challenges face any adolescent, they are often more daunting for those with ADD due to the chronic faulty judgment, impulsiveness, exaggerated need for attention, and social immaturity.

Poor grades, failed tests and classes, disinterest in school—truancy   Failure in school leads to disinterest and avoidance, skipping school, and eventual expulsion or quitting school before graduation. Many adolescents are tired of school and think they are ready for independent life, but the ADD adolescent who has not learned very much in school is particularly unprepared for the challenges awaiting him.

Depression because of poor self-image   It is hard to maintain a positive self-image when confused, failing in school, and not making it socially at a time when success and image can be extremely important. Many adolescents with ADD continue having the low self-esteem that began much earlier in the process.

Increased defiance, anger, and rebelliousness
Lack of success with school and peers can make parents or teachers lay down the law, leading to a response of anger, defiance, and acting out in opposition to authority. Impulsive acts of rebellion make the ADD adolescent feel like he has some control over his own life, when he is actually failing to cope with increasingly challenging demands for performance and self-control.

Destructive behaviors   Frustration and anger can lead the adolescent with ADD to lash out against objects and people. Breaking things, having car accidents, and being abusive or violent to friends and family can cause physical and emotional damage that is irreparable.

Drug and alcohol abuse   Some adolescents will abuse drugs or alcohol to try to self-medicate themselves into better functioning or hedonistic oblivion. Already spaced out, drugs are the last thing that these teenagers need. The stimulant drugs and amphetamines used to treat ADD may be abused for a high or used in smaller doses to temporarily help ADD symptoms. Ritalin is quite popular as a street drug, abused dangerously by snorting it for a high. Alcohol, hallucinogens, opiates, and barbiturates may be used for stimulation or to numb the pain of adolescent struggles. Many of these substances are addictive, leading to long-term problems.

Difficulties or failure in jobs   Teenagers with ADD in their first jobs may meet with disappointment as they are unable to focus and concentrate on complex tasks, having to settle for simpler jobs such as pizza delivery and convenience store clerking. Lack of attention, poor attendance, and impulsive decisions may make even those jobs hard to keep.

Need for constant stimulation   Bored easily, the ADD adolescent needs constant stimulation, often in the form of loud music and videos. Print is much too slow and unstimulating for them. Fast-moving multimedia and computer and video games hold their attention for hours, while slow-moving classroom teaching, books, and magazines are largely ignored. These kids crave change.

Continued restlessness and impulsivity   Restlessness tends to decrease as adolescence turns into adulthood, but impulsivity is often a persistent problem.

Isolation and limited social skills   The social problems of ADD are compounded by extreme peer pressure and awakening sexuality. Where social cues are often subtle, and it is so easy to feel teased and excluded, the ADD teenager often finds herself on the outside of her social circle looking in, without friends or dates. ADD adolescents are often at a loss to know what to do in social situations in which they are already considered to be too spaced out or obnoxious to be acceptable.

Awkwardness in sports   Often physically uncoordinated, teenagers with ADD may never receive the social and personal benefits of excelling in sports and games.

Special Challenges for ADDults

Difficulty with work and career   When adults with ADD eventually get jobs and embark upon a career, challenges often increase. The pressures of deadlines, tardiness, failure to do the work, spacing out on the job, and impulsively talking or acting inappropriately in the workplace often create a pattern of repetitive failure and eventual dismissal. The job history of individuals with ADD often shows a succession of jobs lasting a short time, with an increasing sense of frustration about never fitting in or finding the right career.

Low self-esteem   The net effect of years of inattention, poor achievement, and hyperactivity with the resulting feelings of failure, continual punishment, and disapproval by others can be devastating. Never being able to keep up academically can be quite damaging to one's aspirations, morale, and career potential.

Limited social skills   Socially immature and inappropriate, many ADD sufferers fail to establish and maintain satisfying relationships. All of these factors and more can cause extreme frustration, depression, anxiety, and low self-esteem for these people even though they may be highly intelligent and well-intentioned. They may change partners or get divorced frequently.

Difficulty with reading, learning, concentration, and memory   As the demands of adult life increase, the ability to read, write, focus, and learn new tasks is increasingly difficult for the ADD adult. Their academic deficits catch up with them as they find themselves performing mental tasks less skillfully than the other adults with whom they are competing in the marketplace.

Losing things—forgetting to complete daily tasks
Adults continue to lose and forget important objects and tasks, often leading to disappointment and disapproval from others. Learning organizational skills and using memory aids can bring some order to their world and help them function more normally.

Absentmindedness and daydreaming   Earth is still trying to contact Johnny years later. Adults often continue to be drifty, dreamy, and spacy, and often have to be startled into perceiving the outside world again after a daydreaming interlude.

Seek out constant stimulation and change   Changing jobs, changing relationships, traveling, and non-stop media input are attempts to combat boredom with distraction. This is a lifelong attribute of the ADD personality.

Need for immediate gratification   As part of the boredom syndrome, they need to get immediate return for their actions or they will move on to something else. ADD people are in the moment, without much thought for the future. Now is the only time that seems to exist. "Later" is hard for them to grasp.

Continued restlessness and impulsivity   ADDults are less restless and sometimes less impulsive than their younger counterparts. Maturity counts for something as they settle down and consider their actions more carefully.

Anger and frustration   The frustration and anger that have been building from childhood frequently manifest in the words and actions of adults with ADD. All of the characteristics we have mentioned cause difficulties in life, and anger is a frequent response to these cumulative, unalterable stumbling blocks, as well as the petty but constant frustrations of everyday life with ADD.

3

―――⚭―――

An Epidemic of ADD or a Matter of Overdiagnosis?
Does ADD Really Exist?

Thomas Armstrong, Ph.D., in his controversial book *The Myth of the ADD Child,* insists that ADD is a diagnosis aimed at forcing children to behave in a particular, narrowly defined manner.[2] He claims that children have different learning styles, respond to stress in various ways, and that the condition has been radically overdiagnosed and overtreated. He encourages a wide variety of non-drug interventions including adjustment of the classroom setup, more kinesthetic learning, project-based learning, martial arts classes, visualization, and meditation.

A similar viewpoint is held by Peter Breggin, M.D., author of *Toxic Psychiatry and The War Against Children.* Dr. Breggin, a psychiatrist who refuses to prescribe Ritalin for his patients diagnosed with ADD, holds a strong belief that there is no evidence that symptoms associated with ADD constitute a diagnosis or a mental disorder. He voices

[2] Thomas Armstrong, Ph.D., *The Myth of the ADD Child* (New York: Dutton, 1995).

strong concerns about the possibly damaging long-term effects of Ritalin.[3]

Still a third health professional, child psychiatrist Dr. Stanley Greenspan, writes in his book *The Challenging Child* that a number of attention problems are due to visual, auditory, motor, and spacial processing difficulties. Children with all of these individual difficulties, according to Dr. Greenspan, are often misdiagnosed with ADD.[4]

As homeopathic physicians, we do not believe that it is helpful to lump so many people with widely differing symptoms into one syndrome and treat them all with similar drugs. Having seen several hundred children with mild to major behavioral, learning, and attitudinal problems, we believe that these children need to be handled as individuals with unique problems rather than treated stereotypically. We also favor a treatment approach, homeopathy, that lasts for months or years, not just a few hours.

What About Neurotransmitters?

Most physicians and mental health professionals attribute ADD to an imbalance in transmitters within the brain, often serotonin or dopamine. Many studies have attempted to correlate ADD with specific neurotransmitter abnormalities. A group of researchers from the University of Georgia reviewed these neuroanatomical, neurochemical, and neurophysiological theories and studies.[5] They concluded

---

[3] The Merrow Report, op.cit.

[4] Stanley, Greenspan, Ph.D., *The Challenging Child* (Reading, MA: Addison-Wesley, 1995).

[5] C.A. Ricco *et al.*, "Neurological Basis of Attention Deficit Hyperactivity Disorder," *Exceptional Children*, 60 (1993): 118–124.

that although there is evidence of neurological differences in children diagnosed with ADD, no definitive mechanism has been found for these differences. The authors recommended a differential diagnosis of ADD, learning disability, and conduct disorder. They suggest that it may be more accurate to view the syndrome as a cluster of various behavioral deficits, including attention, hyperactivity, and impulsivity, which share a common response to psychostimulants. Even if neurotransmitters are found definitely to play a role in ADD, homeopaths view such abnormalities as a *result* of a fundamental imbalance of the person as a whole rather than the cause of ADD.

An Overstimulated Society

One correlation which is clear to us is the increasingly rapid pace of our highly technological society and a growing number of children diagnosed with ADD. We live in an extremely overstimulated society. Children spend hours playing Nintendo rather than romping through the woods or playing outside. Many are glued to the television set. Movies are speedier, scarier, and more violent than ever before. There is a growing atmosphere of hurriedness, intensity, and urgency. We eat fast, play fast, and channel-surf. We eat in fast-food restaurants known to decorate their premises in jangly colors so that their customers will eat quickly and move on to make space for the next shift. People look for caffeine and drugs of all kinds to make them go faster and stay up longer. They buy double espressos to pick them up more quickly. They use highly caffeinated amphetamine-like herbs, including ma huang and guarana, that contain seven times as much caffeine as coffee. Our society places little value on tranquillity, quiet, solitude, and the simple joy of being in nature.

Biofeedback is one method to induce deep relaxation by altering brain waves through selective reinforcement. Some have found biofeedback to be helpful for ADD, but the need for frequent treatments may put it economically out of reach for many children and adults.

Is ADD a Dietary Problem?

Parents often tell us that their child's behavior is considerably worse the morning after Halloween or after any sugar binge. Their perceptions have recently been supported by researchers at the Yale University School of Medicine. They found that within a few hours after substantial sugar intake, children release large amounts of adrenaline, which causes them to experience shakiness, anxiety, excitement, and concentration problems. Their brain waves also indicated a decreased ability to focus.[6]

As naturopathic physicians with considerable training in nutrition, we are appalled that the per capita intake of sugar is over 130 pounds per year in this country and that children are the worst fast-food junkies. Many of the parents of our ADD child patients are very nutritionally aware and have had their children tested for food and environmental allergens. Those children we have seen, despite eliminating cow's milk, wheat, and other foods from their diets, have not experienced a consistent and significant improvement in behavior or learning. Some parents have tried the Feingold dietary approach, which eliminates foods with natural salicylates, artificial colors,

[6] *Journal of Pediatrics,* February, 1996 cited in *Well Being Journal,* May/June 1996.

our clinical experience have shown that the Feingold diet has helped only   some children with ADD.[7] In those cases where allergies and sensitivities to additives are a major problem, it is helpful to remove or restrict them. A healthy diet which emphasizes whole, natural foods is likely to benefit the health of any child or adult with ADD and is a useful part of the total treatment plan.

Yet both in examining the scientific literature concerning diet and ADD and in interviewing parents of children with ADD, we have found correlations between ADD and sugar consumption, ingestion of food additives and colorings, and food allergies, and hypoglycemic and anti-yeast diets, to affect some children and not others. We have not found that changing a child's diet has nearly as consistent, profound, and lasting impact on behavioral and learning problems as homeopathic treatment. Dietary approaches undoubtedly do work for some children, but not for many others. We admit that children who have enjoyed a great improvement in behavior strictly from dietary change are not likely to turn up in the office of a homeopath unless their dietary measures stop working and the parents seek out an alternative other than dietary intervention.

Is the Diagnosis of ADD Just A Way to Control the Classroom?

How true are criticisms like those of Drs. Armstrong and Breggin that the overdiagnosis of ADD is a means for teachers and parents to stultify children's freedom and individuality? It is true that some teachers are exces-

---

[7] E.H. Wender, "The Food Additive-Free Diet in the Treatment of Behavior Disorders: A Review," *Developmental and Behavioral Pediatrics* 7 (1986):35–42.

individuality? It is true that some teachers are excessively rigid and wish to run their classrooms like a military academy.

These are the same teachers who bring the parents of any unruly child in for a conference and put pressure on them to put their children on stimulant medications. It is also true that many classrooms have more children than the teacher can possibly handle, and that some of these children are frighteningly violent and exhibit an antipathy to learning. However, other teachers sincerely wish to create more relaxed learning environments in which imagination and creativity are fostered. They, too, often find a growing number of restless, disruptive children who find it next to impossible to concentrate.

Try telling the parent of a child with full-blown ADD, who has tried every possible learning style including home schooling, that the diagnosis is all in the mind of the child's teacher and that her child just needs a less structured learning environment. That parent may look at you in disbelief, insist that her child live with you for a week, and then see what you think.

Gifted or Hyperactive?

One group of children that may be included in the diagnostic category of ADD but which has very specific needs is precocious children with ADD-like symptoms. If you had an IQ of 150 and a photographic mind, how would you feel about being in a regular fourth-grade classroom? You would probably be bored to tears unless your teacher created special activities and outlets for your unusual intellectual capabilities. You might tap your pencil on your desk, design paper skyscrapers, or invent a magical world of dinosaurs. Then when the teacher called on you . . . oops! Sounds a lot like Calvin and Hobbes.

James Webb and Diane Latimer address this dilemma: "In the classroom, a gifted child's perceived inability to stay on task might be related to boredom, curriculum, mismatched learning style, or other environmental factors. Gifted children may spend from one-fourth to one-half of their regular classroom time waiting for others to catch up—even more if they are in a heterogeneously grouped class."[8] They point out that because a gifted child may demonstrate ADD-like behaviors in some settings and not others, one classroom teacher may diagnose her with ADD while the other teachers do not. The authors recommend individual evaluation followed by appropriate curricular and instructional changes to account for advanced knowledge, diverse learning styles, and various types of intelligence. Such individual evaluation is exactly what homeopathy has to offer.

Like Parent, Like Child

We have seen many children who are the spitting image of their parents. They may share one or both parents' behavioral and learning styles. We often hear that the mother or father also had difficulty with reading or concentration, but was never diagnosed as having ADD and somehow made it through school. We have seen little boys with the same explosive tempers and total lack of patience as their type A fathers. We have also seen many a child whose restlessness and inability to concentrate ran through all of the siblings in the family. You will see

[8] James T. Webb and Diane Latimer, "ADHD and Children Who are Gifted," *ERIC Digest*, #E522, 1993.

this phenomenon reflected in some of our case histories later in the book.

Many experts have documented a hereditary aspect to ADD. We saw one child whose chief problem was absentmindedness in spite of intellectual brilliance. All he wanted to do was to read about atoms and quarks and to contemplate the boundlessness of the universe. His father was the same way: brilliant, but he could barely remember to change his socks. His father's father was a renowned educator who had had a number of car accidents because he couldn't be bothered to keep his car on the road. They were like carbon copies of each other.

Yet we see other children whose tantrums, violence, and excessive restlessness seem to come out of nowhere. They may have very mellow parents who have limited their children's exposure to guns, sugar, and violent movies and who have raised them in a very loving, safe environment—and they still behave like wildcats.

A Matter of Predisposition

Even if they have two parents with ADD and eat sugar all day, some children will develop ADD and others will not. What can account for this disparity? Homeopaths believe that the reason some children and adults suffer from ADD and others do not lies in susceptibility. If you ask the parent of a child with ADD when he first noticed problem behaviors or tendencies in his child, he will likely say from infancy or toddlerhood. Such a child may have been hyperalert and have tendencies to wake frequently during the night, to be fussy and hard to satisfy, to run as soon as he could walk, and to climb all over the furniture as soon as he was mobile. This predisposition to ADD-like behavior often occurs at a very tender age. Homeopaths frequently observe that this predisposition or susceptibility depends on the constitution of the individual from birth and may even be affected by the state of the parents prior to conception and during pregnancy.

How is this susceptibility passed on? Genetically? Homeopaths recognize these common traits among parents and children and hypothesize that there is some mechanism which we do not yet understand for these impressions or threads to be passed on generationally. Researchers at the University of California, Irvine recently reported finding the first abnormal gene associated with ADD. The gene controls dopamine receptors in the brain. Children with a more severe form of ADD have an abnormality of this gene, causing less sensitivity to dopamine, a neurotransmitter. Ritalin is known to stimulate dopamine release, perhaps accounting for the drug's efficacy.[9]

Most important to the homeopath are the unique tendencies or predispositions of the individual child or adult, regardless of what specifically may trigger the susceptibility. The phenomenon of susceptibility varies from individual to individual and cannot be stereotyped. But the individual can be carefully listened to and deeply understood. And from this understanding, a homeopathic medicine can be matched to the individual which will shift that susceptibility and bring the person into balance.

No Single Cause of ADD

Our conclusion, which is not particularly surprising given that we are homeopaths, is that each child or adult

---

[9]"Study Links Gene Abnormality to Hyperactive Children," *Seattle Times*, May 1, 1996.

with ADD is individual. The cause of his ADD is no more stereotypical than his symptoms. Other than saying that anyone with ADD must have a predisposition to it, be it hereditary or environmental, we believe it is fruitless to ascribe all of the individual ADDs to one causative factor.

4

---cᗉ᠑᠑᠂---

"MY Child Has ADD?"
Once Your Child Has Been Diagnosed

It can be a shock to have your child diagnosed with ADD. You may feel angry and wonder if the teacher overreacted or dislikes your child. This tends to be a concern especially if the child did well in his previous classroom but now receives poor grades and bad reports concerning academic achievement and/or conduct. If your child acts differently at home than at school, you may feel confused about the diagnosis. Or you may not be too surprised at the diagnosis if you are already aware of your child's difficulties completing homework, paying attention, and following instructions. The diagnosis of ADD can come as a relief. You may feel better if you can apply a label to your or your child's problems.

Your may initially feel very concerned about your child's further abilities to learn, achieve, have a productive livelihood, get along with others, and be happy. You may wonder whether your child's problem is hereditary and whether your other children will also be diagnosed with ADD. You may wonder if you could have been a better parent. You may worry that your child will fail in school due to his ADD. You may worry that he cannot keep up with the challenges of a regular classroom or, on the other hand, that his capabilities will be hindered if he is placed in a special classroom due to his diagnosis of ADD. You may also be seriously concerned about the effect of your ADD child on the rest of the family, particularly if his behavior is aggressive or violent. These are all very normal reactions.

Is Diagnostic Testing Necessary?

Many parents are alerted to the possibility that their child may have ADD at a teacher-parent conference or from problem behavior reports sent home from school. The diagnosis is suggested on the basis of the child's classroom behavioral problems or difficulty with reading, writing, tests, or homework. It is often recommended at this point that the child be tested for ADD by a child psychologist. Such testing may be recommended also to adults, although less frequently.

Whether or not you choose to have yourself or your child run through an extensive battery of tests for ADD may depend on which type of treatment you prefer as well as what type of information you are seeking. Some parents need to have their child's ADD confirmed through psychological testing in order to secure placement in special classes or to receive funding for special education.

If you choose to go the conventional route, many physicians will prescribe the same medications, based on symptoms, regardless of whether your child has been formally tested. If you choose the homeopathic course of treatment, it will generally make little difference whether or not your child has been tested. The homeopath will carefully interview you and your child and base the prescription on the unique characteristics of your child rather than the results of psychological testing.

If you think that it is important to you to have the conventional testing done in order to gather all of the information that is possible and to better understand your child's specific strengths and weaknesses, this may be an important step for you. Once your child has been tested, his or her medical record does reflect a psychiatric diagnosis. A confirmed diagnosis of ADD may put more pressure on the parents, from teachers and school counselors, to seek drug treatment for their child.

Where to Go for Help

Parents commonly go to their family physician once their child has been diagnosed with ADD. That physician may prescribe Ritalin or another medication for the child or may refer the child to a psychiatrist or psychologist. A psychiatrist or psychologist specializing in ADD will be more familiar with the particular medication and dosage options. Many parents have qualms about putting their children on drugs, but choose to do so anyway because they are afraid their children's learning might be impaired if they are unmedicated. The popular and medical literature on ADD strongly recommend the use of stimulants and antidepressants. Parents are led to believe that no other options are possible. Many of the children we see had been on conventional medication for ADD, sometimes for five years or more, before the parents heard about homeopathy. In some cases, the parents discontinued the medications due to side effects or because the medications made no significant improvement in the child's symptoms. In other cases the parents or child simply want to try a more natural alternative. We hope that this book will help to educate more parents about the option of homeopathy to treat ADD before they try the conventional medications.

Popular Support Group Emphasizes Conventional Treatment

We generally encourage our patients to get support from other people who have gone through or conquered problems similar to their own. By far the most popular support group for ADD is C.H.A.D.D. (Children and Adults with Attention Deficit Disorder), which has more than 650 local chapters and over 35,000 members.[10] C.H.A.D.D. sponsors lectures and conferences by many well-known experts on the subject. These conferences are an excellent way to learn about the conventional approach to ADD as well as to get practical, behavioral tips. Documentaries have reported that that the Ciba-Geigy pharmaceutical company, which manufactures Ritalin, has contributed significant amounts of money to C.H.A.D.D. for educational purposes.[11] Both Ciba-Geigy and C.H.A.D.D. deny any conflict of interest. C.H.A.D.D. representatives submitted a petition to the Drug Enforcement Agency requesting that federal regulators lift annual production quotas on methylphenidae (Ritalin) because of the increased demand for the drug. This request was denied.[12]

[10] The Merrow Report, op.cit.
[11] Ibid.
[12] Ibid.

C.H.A.D.D. is skeptical of unproven therapeutic approaches to ADD. Its presentations are generally limited to discussion of drug therapies and educational or behavioral techniques. We have found adult ADD groups to be more open to our presentations on homeopathic treatment. Although C.H.A.D.D's reasoning may be to prevent parents and adults from being unwittingly duped by fads, the result is that many people may be deprived of valuable information about legitimate, safe, and effective therapies, such as homeopathy, that have not yet undergone rigorous scientific testing. C.H.A.D.D. is the primary and, in many cases, the only available ADD support group for thousands of parents. We hope that future research on homeopathic treatment for ADD will convince C.H.A.D.D. to include homeopathy in its presentations. In the meantime, we suggest that C.H.A.D.D. create a forum for discussing alternative approaches to ADD, so that parents and adults can judge the usefulness of these treatments for themselves.

5

------- ⟨∞⟩ -------

To Drug or Not to Drug
The Pros and Cons of Conventional Treatment for ADD

Eight Million Children on Stimulants by the Year 2000?

If the current trend continues, eight million children will be medicated with amphetamines for ADD in the United States by the turn of the century.[13] Since the therapeutic effect of these medications lasts approximately four hours, children need a dose in the morning before leaving for school and another at lunchtime. Children stand in line in the nurse's office or school office to receive their dose of stimulant medication. Steve Friedman, principal since 1990 of Nova Middle School in Fort Lauderdale, Florida, expressed surprise at the growing number of children in his school who were taking Ritalin. When he joined the school, the nurse handed out two prescriptions per day; by 1995 the number had risen to sixty.[14] Given limited school district budgets which limit adequate funding to hire school nurses, doling out

---

[13] The Merrow Report, op.cit.
[14] Ibid.

Ritalin pills is now often written into the job description of school secretaries.

Why Prescribe Speed for ADD?

Although a comprehensive treatment plan for ADD may include behavior modification, cognitive therapy, family therapy, and social skills training, the mainstay of conventional treatment of ADD is medication, usually stimulant medication such as Ritalin (methylphenidate), Dexedrine (dextroamphetamine), Desoxyn (methamphetamine) or Cylert (pemoline). When stimulants are not effective, children may be given tricyclic antidepressants. Stimulants have a short-term effectiveness of 60 to 80 percent in reducing the hyperactivity, distractibility, and impulsiveness of school-age children.[15] Similar rates of success have been found in adults with ADD.[16] Stimulant medications have also been shown to improve attention span, gross motor coordination, impulsivity, aggressiveness, handwriting, and compliance.[17] Short-term learning benefits have been achieved with these medications, but no lasting improvement in academic success has been shown.

A compilation of all the review studies published over the last twenty years on the effects of stimulant medication for ADD showed that what should be expected with medication was temporary management of diagnostic symptoms including overactivity, inattention, and impulsivity, as well as increased compliance, effort,

---

[15] A.R. Adesman and E.H. Wender, "Helping the Hyperactive Child," *Patient Care,* March 30, 1992, 96–116.

[16] Paul H. Wender, *Attention Deficit Hyperactivity Disorder in Adults* (New York/ Oxford: Oxford University Press, 1995), 166.

[17] Adesman and Wender, op. cit., 105.

and academic productivity and decreased aggression and negative behaviors.[18]

School teachers, counselors, and mental health professionals may lean on you to medicate your child and suggest that drugs are "the right thing to do for your child." They may tell you, "If your child had an infection, you would give him antibiotics. So if he has ADD, you need to give him stimulants." Remember, it is your own or your child's health and life that is at stake and you need to feel comfortable about the choice that you make regarding treatment.

Why Think Twice About Prescribing Stimulants?

Many children do respond positively to stimulants, however up to 25 to 40 percent of children with ADD show no response to medication and a large proportion of those who respond to medication respond to a placebo as well.[19] There is no way to predict through physiological, neurological, or biochemical testing who will respond to the medication positively and who will not. The review article showed no significant improvement in reading skills, athletic or game skills, or positive social skills. The improvement in learning and achievement was less than the improvement in behavior and attention. Overall, long-term adjustment, as measured by academic achievement, antisocial behavior, and arrest rate, was unaffected by medication.[20]

---

[18] J.M. Swanson *et al.*, "Effect of Stimulant Medication on Children with Attention Deficit Disorder: A Review of Reviews," *Exceptional Children,* 60 (1993): 154–62.
[19] Ibid., 156.
[20] Ibid., 157.

Furthermore, side effects have been found to occur in some individuals taking stimulant medication. The most commonly occurring side effects are loss of appetite, insomnia, tics (as in Tourette's syndrome), and short-term growth retardation.[21] Some parents report other side effects including headaches, stomach aches, increased heart rate or blood pressure, drowsiness, social withdrawal, irritability and moodiness, and involuntary movements or sounds. Stimulant medication for ADD may be contraindicated for people with seizures, liver disease, heart disease, high blood pressure, or tic disorders.

Studies on the side effects of Ritalin are still inconclusive. Adding to the doubts, the Food and Drug Administration (FDA) just released a study showing that high doses of Ritalin given to mice may cause hepatoblastoma, a rare form of liver cancer. Since there have been no significant reports of liver cancer in children

The Downside of Ritalin

- Derived from the same family as cocaine
- Lasts only four hours
- Treats only some of the symptoms of ADD
- Provides superficial healing, does not treat the root of the problem
- Can cause side effects such as appetite loss, anxiety, insomnia, tics, headaches, stomach aches
- Gets children into the habit of taking drugs
- May need to be taken over entire life span

[21] R.A. Barkley and J.V. Murphy, "Treating Attention-Deficit Hyperactivity Disorder: Medication and Behavior Management Training," *Pediatric Annals,* 20 (1991): 256–66.

taking Ritalin, the FDA still regards the drug as safe and effective.[22]

Most Parents Still Choose Stimulants

Given the lack of consistent long-term benefits, why has stimulant medication continued to be the mainstay of treatment for ADD? Ritalin may have an even greater tendency to relieve stress in the caregiver than in the child.[23] Ritalin and other stimulants do produce significant short-term gains for a large percentage of children and adults with ADD. These gains may be important in preserving the self-esteem of the individual with ADD and the sanity of their teachers, families, and peers. The educational and social benefits of pharmaceutical behavior control are considered far greater than the risks of the medication, and there is no viable alternative available in conventional medicine.

Ritalin as a Recreational Drug

A recently identified drawback of Ritalin is its popularity as an illicit drug. The annual survey "Monitoring the Future" by the University of Michigan warns of a trend concerning Ritalin abuse. From 1993 to 1994 the number of high school seniors admitting to having abused Ritalin doubled, representing about 350,000 students nationwide. Kids call Ritalin "Vitamin-R," "R-ball," or "the

---

[22] "Mother's Little Helper," *Newsweek,* March 18, 1996, 56.
[23] Swanson, op. cit., 156.

smart drug" and seek it out to study better and to get high.[24] A 1995 *Newsweek* article reported that students at an upscale New York college crushed and snorted Ritalin tablets like cocaine. They described an immediate rush, as if they felt hyperactive.[25]

Ritalin consumption has risen nearly sixfold during the past five years.[26] One college student took Ritalin in order to help focus his attention in his studies. Soon he was snorting it twice daily, needing more and more to achieve the same results. The side effects of Ritalin addiction include strokes, hyperthermia, hypertension, and seizures. Several deaths have been attributed to Ritalin abuse, including that of a high school senior in Roanoke, Virginia, who died from snorting Ritalin after drinking beer.[27] According to DEA statistics, emergency room admissions due to Ritalin abuse numbered 1,171 in 1994.[28]

Given the tremendous problem in this country with drug addiction, the growing trend to abuse a drug, which is being legally prescribed for nearly two million children, is of great concern. The manufacturers of Ritalin, in response to the reports of Ritalin abuse, sent pamphlets explaining the proper use of the drug to more than 200,000 physicians and pharmacists.[29]

---

[24] "Ritalin Finding Its Way Into the Schoolyard," *Seattle Times,* February 9, 1996.
[25] "A Risky Rx for Fun," *Newsweek,* October 30, 1995, 74.
[26] Ibid.
[27] Ibid.
[28] *Seattle Times,* February 9, 1996.
[29] "Misuse of Ritalin by Schoolchildren Prompts Warning," *Seattle Times,* March 27, 1996.

An Alternative to Stimulants and Antidepressants

Based on our clinical experience and the reported cases of other homeopathic physicians, homeopathy offers an effective alternative to stimulants and antidepressants in the treatment of ADD. We believe that our clinical results, even more than our experience or opinions, speak for themselves. If even a small percentage of children currently taking stimulants can enjoy instead the long-term, deep-acting benefits of homeopathy, this book will have served its purpose. For those of you who are satisfied with having your children on stimulant medication, we are not trying to prove you wrong. For those of you who are skeptical of homeopathy or of any other alternative to stimulants and other conventional medications in the treatment of children diagnosed with ADD, please read this book before making your decision. For those of you who are unwilling to even consider any treatment that has not been proven by scientific research, no such studies have yet been conducted, but we have received a grant for such a project and hope that you will find the results convincing.

6

Different Strokes for Different Folks

What Parents and Children Say About Drugs for ADD

A Matter of Mixed Reactions

As with any medications, some people are satisfied using Ritalin for ADD and some are not. Some laud the success of Ritalin, others complain of the side effects, and still others complain that their stimulant-medicated children are no longer themselves. The following reactions are of children medicated with Ritalin for ADD whom we have treated with homeopathic medicine, and of their parents. We have tried to include varying points of view, though most of the patients we have quoted are biased in the sense that they sought a more natural alternative to stimulant medication.

"I Still Have That Prescription in My Purse"

"When Michael started having problems in school and the teachers and counselors suggested ADD, we took him to his regular pediatrician. After a forty-five-minute examination, the doctor proclaimed that he was indeed hyperactive and wrote a prescription for twenty milligrams of Ritalin every morning. I can tell you that I still have that prescription in my purse because I just couldn't believe it. We asked about diet, about allergies, about a different form of discipline. Each time the response was the same: 'Ritalin.'

"For some reason it seems to me that our society has come to a point where everyone thinks that you just have to take a pill and whatever problem you have will get better. I just couldn't see giving my child a prescription that ultimately altered his personality. Michael has always been a kind, loving, generous, helpful child. He just doesn't sit still very well at times. I love Michael as he is and I didn't want a pill to change him."

"It Literally Saved Our Lives"

"If Rich had not been given Ritalin at age seven, I don't even care to imagine where or how bad off he would be today. It literally saved our lives! First of all, Rich's reaction to Ritalin gave us the confirmation we needed that there was indeed something physically different about him. Within fifteen minutes after receiving his first dose, we could actually witness him calming down. He could sit still, he could focus, he could carry on a real conversation. He felt good about himself and about life—not high as some people are on speed, but just 'normal' for the first time ever. His social relationships and anger were also improved.

"However, after a few months the side effects of this drug also became difficult to handle. Ritalin did not stay in Rich's system for a predictable length of time. When it wore off, he crashed. We were then given Dexedrine to take along with the Ritalin. The Dexedrine is a time release capsule, so it was longer lasting. But, if he took it alone, it left Rich almost too calm. The Ritalin sort of gave him his life back. Together these medicines worked well for Rich for almost two years. Then he was diagnosed with Tourette's syndrome, which manifested itself in tics and twitches. These were made worse by the Ritalin and eventually he had to discontinue the Dexedrine as well."

None of the Conventional Medications Worked

"Jared is irritable, defensive, and highly offended. He is obsessive about all kinds of things and doesn't show a lot of common sense. He doesn't think before he does things. He has a very hard time in the classroom focusing if something else is going on. He is very intense and interrupts all the time. He is easily touched. Sentimentality and rage are both very close to the surface.

"We tried Ritalin, Cylert, and Prozac. None of them worked. Ritalin made him very frantic and racing and kept him up until two in the morning on even the smallest dose. He became very weepy. With Prozac, he had absolutely no initiative. That's why we're bringing him now to you to try homeopathy." (Quotes from a mother whose child just began homeopathic treatment.)

Ritalin Rebound

"Clay, thirteen, has been on Ritalin for seven years. Because of hormonal changes during puberty, each dose only lasts three hours. What Ritalin does to Clay after he has been off the medication and goes back on is frightening—the tears, the anger. It's that chemical adjustment, like falling off a mountain. The rebound symptoms are worse than when he's off Ritalin entirely. When we tried to stop the medicine for a period of time, it took him four to six weeks to readjust. He had real problems with appetite from the Ritalin. If I wouldn't time the dose and a meal just right, he'd skip a whole meal. Now he just has less of an appetite because of the Ritalin but doesn't skip meals. Other rebound symptoms are headaches and stomach aches.

"Dexedrine also causes a rebound effect with Clay. It lasts only four to six weeks then, if we try to increase the dosage, he becomes terribly angry and unmotivated."

When we asked Clay how he felt about taking Ritalin, he replied, "I don't like it. I have to wait to eat. I need to leave class to take my medicine and it messes up my sports because sometimes I have too much energy and other times too little."

"Ritalin Worked Really Well Sometimes— Sometimes Not"

"Brad has trouble paying attention. Without Ritalin and before he was under homeopathic treatment, he became hyper. Brad had a terrible time paying attention and filtering out the environment. He was constantly asking "What did they say?" He had no restraint. He would eat a whole pack of gum or a sack of candy in one day. He was either very sweet or very awful. There were days when he was easy to get along with and others when he became frustrated and angry, and you couldn't reason with him. He can just get higher and higher and higher.

"Ritalin worked really well sometimes; sometimes not. We wanted to try a more natural treatment so that Brad would have fewer ups and downs."

Jeremy and Krissy

"Jeremy was the perfect child while he was on Ritalin. If you could package a little boy who was polite and sweet, that's how he would be. But he still had trouble concentrating in school. He wouldn't forget things and he got along great with other kids. It was a nightmare when he stopped taking it for a few days or it wore off . . . a rebound. After taking Ritalin for five years, Jeremy developed tics. Now, several years later, he still has them. The tics started like shivers. When the tics are bad, Jeremy is so embarrassed that he doesn't even want to go to school. We tried him on four different stimulant and antidepressant drugs but they didn't work for him. They wanted to try Prozac, but I said no. I didn't want a child of six on Prozac. I don't think I'd ever put him back on Ritalin.

"The same is true with my daughter Krissy. She developed five different side effects from Ritalin. She couldn't gain weight. She looked like a skeleton . . . like a stick figure or someone with anorexia. She was on Ritalin for three years and didn't gain weight until we took her off of it. She also chewed her nails to the quick. Nailbiting is a side effect of Ritalin in some children, you know. Krissy's anxiety level got really high from the drug, too. She would start worrying at eleven in the morning whether she would miss her school bus at three in the afternoon. She got so anxious that she laid out her toothbrush and clothes before going to bed. Sleep was another problem. While she was on Ritalin Krissy didn't want to go to sleep at night.

"We discontinued the medicine a few months ago and now we want to try homeopathy since it has helped her brother."

"It's Not the Real You. It's a Fake Person"

Not all children with ADD feel better on Ritalin. John Merrow interviewed four teenagers who clearly did not want to continue taking Ritalin.[30] They complained, "It's not the real you. It's a fake person. It's totally not me." One of the boys had discontinued the medication by his own choice. A second had been on Ritalin for seven years and begged his parents not to make him take it, but one of his teachers would not allow him in her classroom unless he had a note signed by the school nurse that he had received his Ritalin at school that day. The boys complained of dizziness, stomach upset, inability to sleep, a buzzed feeling, and appetite loss as a result of taking Ritalin.

[30] The Merrow Report, op. cit.

PART TWO

Homeopathy

A Whole
Person Approach

7

Natural Medicine That Works
All About Homeopathy

What Is Homeopathic Medicine?

Homeopathy is a unique form of medicine that comes from different roots than conventional medicine. It was developed as a response to the so-called "heroic" healing methods of eighteenth-century Europe which included the use of toxic substances such as mercury and arsenic in large doses, as well as purging, vomiting, bloodletting, and leeches. Samuel Hahnemann (1755–1843), a brilliant German physician, chemist, and medical translator, was a harsh critic of the methods of his day and strove to find a rational alternative that followed the healing principles of nature. Fluent in at least seven languages, Hahnemann extensively studied the ancient and current medical literature in order to discover what he believed to be the true principles of healing.

Two Paradoxes

Hahnemann's two principal discoveries were the Law of Similars and the idea of using microdoses, extremely tiny doses of medicine, to stimulate the body's ability to heal itself. Both of these discoveries are inherently paradoxical.

The Law of Similars states that a substance from nature that has the ability to *cause* a set of symptoms in a healthy person can *cure* those same symptoms in a sick person. The substance that produces the most similar symptoms will heal most effectively. Using toxic or poisonous substances for healing is paradoxical, but Hahnemann found them to work quite effectively when used in the right way. Poisons kill, or poisons cure, depending on how you use them.

Hahnemann first discovered the Law of Similars during his experiment to discover why quinine (the active substance in today's conventional antimalarial drugs), extracted from Peruvian Cinchona bark, cured malaria. The accepted explanation that it cured because it was bitter did not satisfy Hahnemann since he was aware of many other bitter herbs which did not cure malaria. Hahnemann took repeated doses of the extract himself to see what would happen. He developed periodic chills and fever, common symptoms of malaria. He reasoned that the bark was effective in treating malaria because it could produce symptoms similar to the disease.

He went on to test over 100 substances on himself and his students to discover what symptoms they would produce. Applying the results of his findings in his clinical practice, he found that this new form of medicine successfully treated a significant number of patients with acute and chronic diseases which up to that time had been considered incurable.

Many of the physicians of Hahnemann's time were favorably impressed with his ideas and experiments, and especially with his clinical results in treating mental and emotional as well as physical illnesses. Homeopathy spread rapidly in the early nineteenth century and became renowned for its effectiveness in treating epidemic diseases such as cholera, malaria, typhoid, yellow fever, and scarlet fever.

Weaker Is Stronger

In order to accomplish healing without significant side effects, Hahnemann realized that the substance dose must be very small. Large doses were effective based on the Law of Similars, but their toxic side effects made them less appealing as medicines. He created small doses by repeatedly diluting the original substance in a water and alcohol mixture to remove the toxicity and create a safe, effective medicine. Hahnemann found, however, that if he diluted the medicines too much, their effectiveness was lost. He learned to retain the effectiveness of the medicine and to actually make it stronger by performing *succussion* (a process of shaking the medicine in order to evenly distribute the liquid). He called the combined process of serial dilution and succussion *potentization.*

Homeopaths commonly use medicines made with 30, 200, 1,000, or 10,000 dilutions, far exceeding the point at which molecules of the original substance should remain in the solution. How is this possible? No one really knows how the information pattern in homeopathic medicines persists during dilution beyond the disappearance of the physical molecules of the original substance. This has caused skepticism and prejudice about homeopathy in scientific circles, because the mechanism which preserves the pattern through the potentization process is unknown. Theories have been suggested that polarized molecules such as those in alcohol or water are capable of forming liquid crystals that "remember" the pattern of the original substance.

Homeopathic medicines produce very different effects depending on the original substance from which they were derived. Even at very high dilution factors, each medicine retains its unique characteristics and the ability to dramatically affect people's health. Some factor must persist at high dilutions that is responsible for the clinical success of homeopathic medicines. We look forward to additional scientific research which will confirm the precise mechanism of just how homeopathy works. A recently published book, *Homeopathy: A Frontier in Medical Science,* gives a good review of these controversial issues, as well as current research on homeopathic medicine.[1]

Is There Research on Homeopathy?

Double-blind clinical studies have shown the effectiveness of homeopathic medicine as compared with a placebo in research on common medical conditions. A 1991 review of over 100 homeopathic research studies published between 1966 and 1990 showed that homeopathy showed positive results in 76 percent of the studies in conditions including infections, digestive disorders, influenza, hay fever, rheumatoid arthritis, fibromyalgia, recovery from surgery, and psychological problems. The authors concluded that they could not account for the positive results, but that further research with improved

[1] Paolo Bellavite and Andrea Signorini, *Homeopathy: A Frontier in Medical Science* (Berkeley: North Atlantic, 1995).

methodology was warranted.[2] A recent study, published in 1994 by the peer review journal *Pediatrics* by Jennifer Jacobs, M.D., and associates, demonstrated homeopathy's effectiveness in pediatric diarrhea in Nicaragua.[3] The most recent major study was published in the prestigious British journal *The Lancet*. Scottish researchers David Taylor Reilly and his associates found that 82 percent of asthma sufferers who were treated with homeopathic dilutions of their main allergens improved significantly as compared to the 38 percent improvement in the placebo control group.[4]

Unfortunately, lack of funding has stymied scientific study of the homeopathic treatment of ADD. We were asked to participate in one such study, but the federal funding did not materialize. We would be extremely eager to participate in a sound, well-designed study, and hope that this book paves the way for such research opportunities. Homeopaths have always, and continue to, base their evidence for the effectiveness of homeopathy on clinical results with many patients. These results are shared in professional homeopathic journals and case conferences. It is unfortunate that the scientific community still holds research as the only measure of validity of any treatment modality, because clinical evidence of the effectiveness of homeopathic treatment of ADD speaks for itself.

[2] J. Kleijnan, P. Knipschild, and G. ter Riet, "Clinical Trials of Homeoepathy," *British Medical Journal*, February 9, 1991, 302:316–23.
[3] Jacobs, L., M Jimenez, S. Gloyd, and D. Crothers, "Treatment of Acute Childhood Diarrhea with Homeopathic Medicine: A Randomized Clinical Trial in Nicaragua," *Pediatrics*, May 1994, 93, 5:719–25.
[4] David Reilly, Morag Taylor, Neil Beattie, *et al.*,"Is Evidence for Homeopathy Reproducible?" *The Lancet*, December 10, 1994, 344:1601–6.

Homeopathy Remains Controversial

It may initially be difficult to grasp the idea of home-opathy; that substances that cause symptoms can also cure them, and that tiny doses work even if they are diluted past the point where the substance physically disappears. Some people encountering these facts about homeopathy consider them to be impossible. How then does one account for the fact that homeopathic medicines have repeatedly demonstrated positive clinical results in controlled studies? The fact that the basis for homeopathy is unknown should not lead to discounting it, but to a greater effort to understand it. Unfortunately, conventional medical science has not yet made an unbiased investigation of homeopathy, mostly due to prejudice and fear of academic ridicule for investigating a taboo subject. Those physicians and scientists who do investigate homeopathy with an open mind often change from critics to proponents.

Is Ritalin Acting Homeopathically?

In conventional medicine, it has been demonstrated repeatedly in controlled studies that stimulants such as Ritalin and Dexedrine improve the symptoms of ADD, but no satisfactory mechanism has been proposed. In *A Parent's Guide to Attention Deficit Disorders,* published in 1991, the author says, "The idea of using a stimulant to treat hyperactivity may seem illogical. After all, according to the literature that accompanies stimulants, they are supposed to increase, not decrease motor activity. High doses of these drugs can indeed have a stimulating affect on normal individuals. . . ." She goes on to say, "How [stimulants] act to reduce overactivity and increase attention in children with ADHD is not fully understood."[5] Using stimulants to help hyperactivity seems contradictory, yet it is a widely accepted fact among physicians and researchers that stimulants work for ADD in the short term. It is simply referred to as "a paradoxical effect." Clinical effectiveness is enough reason for the practicing physician to use these drugs, even when their mechanism of action is unknown. We ask these same individuals who have accepted the paradox of stimulants for ADD to carefully and open-mindedly examine homeopathy, which is also paradoxical yet proven repeatedly to be clinically effective despite its mysterious mechanism.

Could it be that the relative success in using stimulants for ADD is in fact because the physicians have stumbled upon a crude form of homeopathy? If stimulants can produce hyperactivity in healthy people, can they also cure it in those with ADD? If that is the case, what is lacking in conventional treatment with stimulants is the individualization of treatment which homeopathy offers to the patient. Homeopaths choose a single medicine made from a substance which could produce the patient's unique pattern of ADD symptoms, rather than trying to treat all patients with ADD with the same medicine.

What Makes Homeopathy Unique?

Homeopathy is very different from other forms of medicine. Conventional medicine treats with various kinds of drugs, which may interact negatively with each other, or

---

[5] Lisa J. Bain, *A Parent's Guide to Attention Deficit Disorders,* New York: Dell Publishing, 1991, 93.

cause complex combinations of side effects. Homeopathy uses only a single medicine because of the single principle that guides homeopathic practice, the Law of Similars.

The challenge in homeopathy is to pick the one substance from nature that truly matches the patient's symptoms. Rather than giving many different drugs to a patient, a homeopath gives only a single natural medicine that is individualized according to the patient's pattern of symptoms. Homeopaths treat the *patient* not the disease. This means that ten patients with ADD may need ten different homeopathic medicines. Their individual differences are what lead the homeopath to choose a particular medicine that can help each of them lead a happier, better adjusted, more productive life. The homeopathic medicine must match the patient's symptom pattern or picture in order to be effective. When the match is made well and the prescription is correct, the patient will markedly improve physically, mentally, and emotionally.

Although homeopathic medicines are made from substances which can cause symptoms if given too frequently or in too large a dose, in the microdoses used in treatment the medicines are extremely safe. They are largely free from side effects. Some patients may experience a brief initial worsening of their symptoms before getting better, which may last from few hours up to a week or more. Rarely, symptoms that belong to the medicine but were not symptoms of the patient may appear briefly if the dosage is too frequent, but will usually go away readily when the medicine is stopped.

From Tarantulas to Platinum

Homeopathic medicines come from all over the world and from extremely diverse substances. Nearly any substance from nature can be used as a homeopathic medicine. Medicines are made from all three kingdoms: animal, plant, and mineral. Poisonous plants such as digitalis and agaricus muscaria (toxic mushrooms), snake and spider venoms such as rattlesnake and tarantula, milk of mammals such as humans, dogs, and dolphins, and mineral elements and their salts, such as platinum, table salt, and sulphur, are all used as homeopathic medicines. Hidden in each of these substances is a unique pattern of the symptoms people develop when they become ill. A few of the homeopathic medicines which have been used successfully for ADD include tarantula spider (*Tarentula hispanica*), white hellebore (*Veratrum album*), datura stramonium (*Stramonium*), deadly nightshade (*Belladonna*), iodide of arsenic (*Arsenicum iodatum*), zinc (*Zincum metallicum*), and silver nitrate (*Argentum nitricum*). Many other homeopathic medicines can also be used depending on the unique symptoms of the patient.

The secrets of the substances used in homeopathy are unlocked by experiments called *provings,* which were initially done by Hahnemann and his students on healthy volunteers including themselves. In a proving, a substance unknown to the participants or *provers* is given in either a crude dose if its toxicity is not too great or in a homeopathic dilution until they begin to develop symptoms. Provers record whatever happens to them physically, mentally, and emotionally during the experiment. These records are carefully analyzed to determine the symptoms which that particular substance can produce and ultimately cure when made into a potentized homeopathic medicine.

Provings done on the same substance in different parts of the world often yield remarkably similar results, demonstrating the universality of the Law of Similars. All provers do not respond identically to a given substance. Some are more susceptible, others less. One prover may respond with more physical symptoms while another may bring out emotional or mental problems. With a large enough group, however, the full picture of the substance emerges. Provers often report personal health benefits from participating in the proving.

Provings are still being done today. Recent provings have been done on chocolate, hydrogen, dolphin's and lion's milks, lavender, scorpion, tungsten, eagle's blood, neon, Douglas Fir, and other sources, allowing these diverse substances to be used effectively as homeopathic medicines.

Regulation and Availability of Homeopathic Medicines

Homeopathic medicines are regulated by the Food and Drug Administration (FDA) as over-the-counter (OTC) drugs. According to recent information from the American Homeopathic Pharmaceutical Association in Valley Forge, Pennsylvania, sales of homeopathic medicines are currently increasing at a rate of about 20 percent per year. Homeopathic pharmacies must follow rigid guidelines established by the *Homeopathic Pharmacopoeia of the United States*. Some of these medicines are available over the counter in pharmacies or health food stores. Others can only be obtained by licensed medical practitioners. The doses available over the counter are often considerably lower than would be used by a homeopathic physician in the case of ADD. The medicines referred to in this book are always single-substance preparations as opposed to combination homeopathic medicines that are available to treat colds, flus, and other acute conditions if one is not under the care of a homeopath.

Homeopathy Throughout the World

Although homeopathy is just beginning to become well known in the United States, it is widely practiced in the rest of the world. A 1993 study published in the *New England Journal of Medicine* revealed that one-third of all Americans are using some form of alternative medicine and that, in 1990, two and a half million Americans used homeopathy and made nearly five million visits to homeopathic practitioners.[6]

India, England, France, Germany, Mexico, and South America are centers of widespread homeopathic practice. The royal family in England has used and supported homeopathy extensively since 1830. More than twenty homeopathic schools or part-time courses flourish in England, including a course for medical doctors at the Royal London Homeopathic Hospital. The Society of Homeopaths maintains a registry of homeopathic practitioners and 42 percent of British family practitioners refer to homeopaths.[7] Over 11,000 French physicians use homeopathic medicines, which are dispensed by more than 20,000

[6] David M. Eisenberg, Ronald C. Kessler, Cindy Foster, *et al.*, "Unconventional Medicine in The United States," *New England Journal of Medicine*, January 28,1993, 328, 4:246–52.
[7] Richard Wharton and George Lewith, "Complementary Medicine and the General Practitioner," *British Medical Journal*, June 7, 1986, 292: 1498–1500.

pharmacies.[8] Thirty-six percent of French citizens have been treated homeopathically.[9] Homeopathic treatment is reimbursed through the national health care system in France and in a number of other European countries. Excellent postgraduate homeopathic courses are offered widely throughout Europe. India has more than 120 homeopathic medical colleges, and more than 100,000 homeopathic practitioners, a legacy of the British Raj.[10] The United States is behind the times in its acceptance of homeopathy.

[8] Dana Ullman, *Discovering Homeopathy-Medicine for the 21st Century* (Berkeley: North Atlantic Books, 1988), 48.
[9] Dana Ullman, *The Consumer's Guide to Homeopathy* (New York: Tarcher/Putnam, 1996), 36.
[10] Ibid., 39.

8

⸺◦⧓◦⸺

An Alternative to Ritalin
Homeopathy as a Highly Effective
Treatment for ADD

One Diagnosis or Many?

The epidemic proportions of the ADD diagnosis are gaining widespread attention from parents, educators, physicians, and other healthcare providers. Many people are seriously questioning the possibility of overdiagnosis. This issue was raised in an informative cover article in *Newsweek* magazine.[11] "ADHD has become America's No. l childhood psychiatric disorder. . . . Since 1990, Dr. Daniel Safer of Johns Hopkins University School of Medicine calculates, the number of kids taking Ritalin has grown two and a half times. Among today's 38 million children at the ages of five to fourteen, he reports, 1.3 million take it regularly. Sales of the drug last year alone topped $350 million. This is, beyond question, an American phenomenon. The rate of Ritalin use in the United States is at least five times higher than in the rest of the world, according to federal studies."

[11] "Mother's Little Helper," *Newsweek,* March 18, 1996, 50–56.

The article continues, "For all the success they've had in treating ADHD, many doctors are convinced that Ritalin is overprescribed." Dr. Peter S. Jensen, chief of the Child and Adolescent Disorders Research Branch of the National Institutes of Mental Health is quoted: "I fear that ADHD is suffering from the 'disease of the month' syndrome." Dr. Bruce Epstein, a St. Petersburg, Florida, pediatrician, reports that parents of normal children have asked him to prescribe Ritalin just to improve their children's grades. "When I won't give it to them, they switch doctors."[12]

We applaud Dr. Thomas Armstrong's warning about the current overdiagnosis of ADD in his book *The Myth of the ADD Child*. We have seen a number of children who were high-spirited, extremely imaginative, and so precocious that their parents were unable to keep up with their ceaseless questions and insatiable intellectual appetites. We have also met children who were over-amped, but performed just fine in school. Many of these children have been diagnosed with ADD, even though we feel they fall more into the category of unusual, remarkable, or gifted children. Some youngsters are the victims of rigid, overly strict teachers whose highly structured classroom environments simply do not pace their temperaments and learning styles. Or they have excessively rule-bound parents who do not extend to their children the freedom that they need to thrive and expand their creative talents.

We have also seen a large number of children whose behaviors are very disruptive and disturbing through no fault of teachers. No one can expect a teacher in a classroom of forty active children to cope

[12] Ibid., 52.

happily with the statistical average of 10 percent (four children) in her class with ADD. The amount of extra attention, discipline, and time just trying to keep these children and those around them safe is more than many teachers can handle.

Can we, however, lump all of these children together under one diagnostic category? Can a child who lashes out at his family, peers, and teachers in a violent, destructive manner and has no interest in his schoolwork fit into the same diagnostic group as a sweet, gregarious child who simply cannot pay attention in class? Conventional medicine would say that, based on their scores on standardized ADD tests, both children could indeed have ADD. Homeopathy would say that these are two distinct children whose problems and temperaments are as different as night and day. A homeopath would prescribe very different medicines for the two children, rather than giving them both stimulants.

And what about the many conditions that mimic ADD, such as dyslexia and other learning disabilities, vision and auditory problems, epilepsy, developmental disorders, hypothyroidism, hyperthyroidism, hypoglycemia, food allergies, lead poisoning, caffeinism, anxiety, depression, and obsessive compulsive disorder, just to name a few? It is essential to understand and differentiate each individual child, not only from the viewpoint of psychological testing, but also to comprehend deeply the physical symptoms, experience, feelings, beliefs, and motivations of each child.

Unlike many other syndromes there is no physical examination or laboratory test that definitely confirms the diagnosis of ADD. While some psychologists and educators use various scales, others, including physicians, often base the diagnosis on the subjective reports of parents and teachers. The inconsistency of diagnostic criteria and apparent overdiagnosing in this country has led many to question the diagnosis of ADD. Some educational experts acknowledge that "The position that ADHD is not a proven syndrome has many advocates, physicians as well as educators. However, whether or not a syndrome exists, it is clear that many children have difficulty in school because of an inability to attend to tasks. The ideal would be to describe each child's strengths and weaknesses and offer an individualized program."[13] We would like to take this a step further: Offer an individualized medicine as well as a learning program tailored to the needs of the individual child.

The Homeopathic Approach to ADD

Homeopaths are able to treat ADD effectively in many cases by bringing the individual into balance. Homeopaths treat people with ADD, not the ADD itself. For a homeopath, what needs to be treated is the specific pattern of symptoms which an individual presents. Only the one homeopathic medicine that specifically matches the unique symptoms of the individual will allow the person to live in a functional way.

Each of these individuals included in this book is unique, and it is that uniqueness that leads to the homeopathic prescription in such a different way than

---

[13] L. Rebecca Campbell, M.D., and Morris Cohen, Ed.D., "Management of Attention Deficit Hyperactivity Disorder: A Continuing Dilemma for Physicians and Educators," *Clinical Pediatrics,* March, 1990, 29: 191–3.

with conventional medicine. Our clinical experience, presented in the case studies in this book, as well as the published experience of other homeopaths, suggests strongly that homeopathy is a useful treatment for ADD. Homeopaths always take the whole person into account. If the chief complaint of the person is his inability to sit still, difficulty concentrating, or other symptoms of ADD, these behaviors would certainly be taken into account, but in combination with all the person's other symptoms. The homeopath would note anything unusual about that person. That might include a history of scarlet fever during childhood, a strong fear of birds, recurrent dreams of falling out of bed at night and no one coming to the rescue, or a craving for persimmons. The homeopath sincerely seeks to understand the uniqueness of the patient.

The Pros of Homeopathic Treatment of ADD

- Treats the whole person at the root of the problem
- Considered safe, without the side effects of Ritalin and other medications
- Uses natural, nontoxic medicines
- Treats each person as an individual
- Heals physical as well as mental and emotional symptoms
- Lasts for months or years rather than hours
- Is inexpensive
- Is cost-effective

Why Choose Homeopathy over Conventional Medicine for ADD?

• The most common reason patients choose homeopathic treatment is the positive results they have heard from others with similar problems or because they have been referred by another physician or practitioner who is familiar with homeopathic treatment of ADD.

• The patient or parents have read about homeopathy, and the philosophy and approach make more sense to them than conventional medicine.

• Many adults and parents choose homeopathic treatment because it is safe, nontoxic, and effective.

• Conventional medications for ADD act very briefly. A dose of Ritalin, for example, lasts only about four hours. One dose of the correct homeopathic medicine usually lasts at least four to six months.

• Homeopathic medicines often result in growth spurts in children and never suppress a child's normal development. Nor do they cause such side effects as tics, appetite suppression, and insomnia.

• Homeopathic medicines are very inexpensive. The only significant cost of homeopathic treatment is office visits. Once the person has responded well to the homeopathic medicine, appointments are infrequent.

• Homeopathy treats the whole person. Not only do learning and behavioral problems improve, so do most or all of the other physical, mental, and emotional complaints of the person. Conventional medication for ADD works only on specific learning and behavioral problems. Sally Smith, a parent of an ADD child formerly on Ritalin, describes this phenomenon by holding up a ruler and pointing to the one-inch mark: "Ritalin makes you available to learn. You and your parents and teachers have to work on all the rest."[14]

• Homeopathy will not make a child depressed or dull. Parents sometimes complain that, although stimulant and antidepressant medications have eliminated some of the more severe problem behaviors, their children's spirits seem dampened and they do not seem like their former selves.

• Homeopathic medicines are generally given infrequently and over limited periods of time. Conventional medications put only a temporary lid on ADD symptoms. Doctors often recommend that these medications be taken for the rest of the patient's life.

What Can I and My Family Expect from Homeopathic Treatment?

Homeopaths have high expectations for their patients. We generally do not consider a homeopathic medicine effective for a patient unless the person's symptoms are at least 50 percent (usually 70 percent or more) improved and this improvement lasts for a year or more. This requires that the patient stay with homeopathic treatment for at least a year. The homeopath keeps a careful record of all of the symptoms and characteristics that were elicited during each interview. As treatment progresses, these symptoms should get better and better. An improvement can usually be noticed within one month, and often within days or weeks.

A patient can expect his energy and overall sense of well-being to improve as well as an improvement in most or all of his mental, emotional, and physical

---

[14] *Newsweek,* op. cit., p. 56.

complaints. This means, as you will see over and over in the cases that we present in this book, that not only does attention and behavior improve, but headaches, growing pains, constipation, nailbiting, and other symptoms improve after the homeopathic medication has been prescribed.

Can Homeopathic and Conventional Medicines Be Used Together?

This is one of the most common questions we are asked by adults or parents of children who have been diagnosed with ADD. This is ultimately a decision between the patient and the prescribing physician. A general guideline is to assess whether the prescription medication is effective. In cases where the patient sees no improvement from the medication that has already been prescribed, the prescribing physician and patient generally agree to stop the medication and to try homeopathy instead.

In other cases, the medication is working but the side effects are disturbing. With still other patients, the prescription medication is having a positive effect, but the patient or parents do not like the idea of staying on medication and seek a more natural alternative. In these situations, the patient or parents may inform the prescribing physician that they wish to discontinue the medication long enough to try an alternative.

Another category of patients feels that their symptoms of ADD are so severe that they dare not discontinue their medications until they have found another therapy that is effective. In such a case, many homeopaths will prescribe the homeopathic medication in addition to the prescription drugs the person is already taking. As the homeopathic medicine works and the patient improves, the patient can work with his physician to taper off the prescription medication. This process requires knowledge and experience and is another compelling reason to seek an experienced homeopath.

What If My Doctor Does Not Believe in Homeopathy?

From the time that homeopathic medicine was first brought to this country in the early 1800s, there have been many skeptics among medical doctors. Homeopathic philosophy is very different from what is taught in conventional medical schools. When homeopathy is mentioned in a medical history class, it is generally dismissed as an aberration of the past.

With the growing interest in homeopathic medicine and with the disillusionment about the side effects and short-term benefits of much of modern medical treatment, a growing number of conventional doctors are opening their minds to homeopathy. Some medical doctors are incorporating homeopathy into their conventional practices or referring to other homeopathic practitioners. In our practice, we receive many referrals from medical doctors and osteopaths. Many conventionally trained physicians and other licensed healthcare practitioners have studied homeopathy in the courses that we teach through the International Foundation for Homeopathy. Many physicians, although they may know nothing about homeopathy, encourage their patients, especially children, to use any therapies that are of real benefit to that person rather than, or in combination with, conventional medicines.

If your physician or your child's physician is adamantly opposed to you trying homeopathy and it is your choice to do so, you can try to educate him or her about homeopathic treatment of ADD or you can find a physician who is more supportive of your freedom of choice. Homeopathic practitioners are generally happy to educate conventional physicians about homeopathic philosophy and treatment. Even a skeptical person may be convinced of the possible benefits of homeopathy if he or she reads case studies, attends a homeopathic case conference, or sees the results of successful homeopathic treatment.

Using Homeopathy Along with Other Therapies

Homeopathic medicine is very compatible with many other treatment modalities. Family and individual counseling is often much more effective and proceeds more quickly when one or more family members are under homeopathic treatment. When the whole person is in balance, his mind is generally clearer and he is much more able to move forward in his life.

Therapies such as chiropractic, craniosacral, auditory integration, psychotherapy, and biofeedback are fine to pursue along with homeopathy. Once the correct homeopathic medicine has been given, many patients find that they no longer need to follow strict allergy rotation diets, receive desensitization injections, take megadoses of numerous vitamins and minerals, and use other therapies aimed at treating individual symptoms. It is very understandable that individuals with ADD want to try anything that has the possibility of helping them, but using too many therapies, conventional or alternative, at the same time can make it very difficult to discern what effect each specific therapy is having. When a person receives the correct homeopathic medicine, she knows it. She feels an improvement in energy, physical ailments, concentration, attitude, and creativity. Once she feels so much better, she generally no longer needs lots of other therapies.

Are There Any Things I Can't Do During Homeopathic Treatment?

There are certain substances and exposures that consistently interfere with homeopathic treatment. Most practitioners will advise you to avoid the following substances: coffee, eucalyptus, camphor, menthol, recreational drugs, and electric blankets. You will be asked to avoid using topical medications such as topical steroids, antibiotics, antifungals, and to use oral antibiotics and cortisone products only after consulting your homeopath, except in cases of emergency. Acupuncture, although a treatment of tremendous value, is not recommended during homeopathic treatment. Nor are other treatments, which are prescribed in order to remove specific symptoms without treating the whole person.

Can Homeopathy Help Me or My Child?

Most people are potential candidates for homeopathic treatment. As with any treatment, you must make a commitment to follow the recommendations of your homeopath. You must be willing to follow these guidelines:

1. You should stay with homeopathic treatment for a minimum of six months to one year before seeking out other therapies.
2. You, as a patient or a parent or family member, need to provide thorough and honest information to the homeopath. The better the homeopath understands the patient, the more likely the best medicine can be found and a lasting cure can result.
3. You need to inform the homeopath of any medications that you or your child is taking. Once there has been improvement with homeopathic treatment, prescription medications for ADD are generally unnecessary. A growing number of conventional physicians are encouraging parents to seek alternative treatment for ADD in hopes that the children will not need to be medicated throughout childhood and sometimes throughout much of their lives.
4. There are a small number of substances and influences, such as coffee and recreational drugs, which are likely to interfere with homeopathic treatment and which you will need to avoid. Homeopathic practitioners will make their own recommendations regarding this matter.
5. You need to come for scheduled appointments and to inform the homeopath of any significant changes in your health during the course of homeopathic treatment. Homeopathic follow-up appointments are generally every six weeks to three months. Once you are doing well, follow-ups are scheduled less frequently.

The Limitations of Homeopathic Treatment

Homeopathic treatment is not for everyone. The following are factors that prevent a person from being a good candidate for homeopathic treatment:

1. There are some children, particularly teenagers, who are so opposed to anything their parents recommend that they will sabotage homeopathic treatment, either by refusing to go to appointments or take the medicines or by intentionally using substances that interfere with homeopathic treatment. Similarly, both parents need to be convinced that homeopathy is a valid treatment or willing to try it for at least six months.

2. Some people have such severe behavioral problems that they need to be in an institution, such as a jail or drug or alcohol treatment center, rather than outpatient treatment. We are aware of only one such institutional program, which offered homeopathy as part of a research study and hope others will in the near future.[15]

3. Individuals who are unwilling to avoid those substances which interfere with homeopathic treatment, such as coffee or recreational drugs, are not good candidates for homeopathy.

4. Homeopathic medicines may not act as quickly initially as prescription drugs, though the positive effects last much longer. This requires patience and a willingness to stick with the treatment process.

Why Not Treat Yourself or Your Family?

As you read through the cases in this book, you will probably think of someone you know who may have a very similar symptom picture. You may even be tempted to try to find the medicines mentioned in this book and

---

[15] Garcia-Swain, S. "Homeopathy and Drug Abuse: A Review of a Double-blind Trial with 703 Patients," National Center for Homeopathy Conference, May, 1996.

administer them yourselves. Please heed our advice regarding self-treatment.

There are many classes available on prescribing homeopathic medicines for acute illnesses such as colds, flus, and minor infections. We encourage you to take these classes, to read more about acute prescribing, to buy a homeopathic home kit, and to try homeopathic medicines on yourself and your family for minor illnesses. If the person treated does not improve in a day or two, be sure to consult your homeopathic or conventional physician.

The conditions mentioned in this book are not acute conditions. These are chronic states and need to be handled much more carefully. There are over 2,000 homeopathic medicines. It takes years of homeopathic study and practice to make the fine distinctions about when to prescribe which medicine. Although homeopathic medicines do not have long lists of side effects like many conventional medicines, it is also possible to experience a reaction to the medicine. IN ANY CHRONIC CONDITION, WHETHER PHYSICAL, MENTAL, OR EMOTIONAL, DO NOT TREAT YOURSELF OR YOUR CHILD. Find an experienced homeopathic practitioner. We have received a number of calls from people who have read our articles on ADD, thought they recognized themselves or their children, and gone out to find the medicine themselves. Invariably they have called us for treatment because they did not select the right medicine or did not know how to administer the medicine at the right frequency or potency. If you were considering brain surgery, you would not read a book or two, buy a set of scalpels, and start cutting. Homeopathy is just as complicated an art as neurosurgery. Just because homeopathic medicines are widely available does not mean they are easy to use. Please do not experiment on yourself or your family members for ADD. Find an expert.

How Can I Find a Homeopath?

A growing number of health care practitioners, including medical doctors (M.D.), naturopathic physicians (N.D.), osteopathic physicians (D.O.), chiropractors (D.C.), family nurse practitioners (F.N.P.), physicians' assistants (P.A.), acupuncturists (L.A., C.A., or O.M.D.), and veterinarians (D.V.M.), practice homeopathic medicine. Some homeopaths are unlicensed. We know of no experienced homeopaths in the United States who focus solely on patients with ADD. Since a homeopath always treats the whole person, such specialization is not necessary to find good treatment. What is most important is to find a practitioner who specializes in classical homeopathy, who spends at least an hour with each new patient, prescribes one homeopathic medicine at a time based on a detailed interview rather than a machine, and waits at least five weeks before assessing the progress of the patient. If at all possible, find a homeopath who is board certified or very experienced. It is not always possible to find a homeopath in your immediate area, or even your state. You will be likely to find much better results, even if you need to travel or do your homeopathic consultations by telephone, than to go to someone in your area who knows some homeopathy, but is not experienced and does not specialize in homeopathy. We treat many patients by phone, though we prefer to do the initial interview in person if at all possible.

In the appendix you can find the names and addresses of organizations that publish directories of homeopathic practitioners in the United States. It is still wise to speak to the practitioner directly to make sure he or she meets the guidelines we have suggested.

9

Unique Treatment for Unique Individuals
Treating People Not Diagnoses

Understanding the Individual with ADD

One fundamental distinction between conventional medicine and homeopathy is that conventional medicine places a large number of people into a small number of diagnostic categories. It is true that psychiatrists, psychologists, and conventional therapists recognize subgroups of ADD including people with problems with attention, oppositional behavior, and conduct. However, there is a vast difference between the behaviors, personalities, and characteristics of the many individuals that fall under the one diagnostic umbrella of ADD. This diagnosis may include a violent, aggressive child who smashes doors and bites others, as well as a mild-mannered, shy child whose behavior is fine but who has difficulty concentrating. In conventional medicine, these two children will probably both be diagnosed with ADD and both given some form of stimulant or other medication. But there are two extremely different individuals. Their diagnosis of ADD may be the only thing these two people have in common.

The homeopath seeks to deeply understand the state of each individual. There are more than 2,000 homeopathic medicines and each person will benefit most at any given time from the one specific medicine that best matches his symptoms. The homeopath conducts an extensive interview in which she delves into the specific behaviors, feelings, attitudes, beliefs, and motivations of the individual. We not only ask in great detail about the behaviors of the person, but about his dreams, fears, physical symptoms, prenatal and birth history, family medical history, food preferences, sleep position, and much more. The intent is to understand the individual from the inside out; to perceive what makes him tick. It is only through deeply understanding each individual that the homeopath can successfully match one of the 2,000 homeopathic medicines to that particular person.

You may ask how this is different from the interview or testing that a psychiatrist or psychologist might perform in order to determine a conventional diagnosis of ADD. It is a very different process. The homeopath is not interested in labels but in the uniqueness of each person. Conventional testing groups individuals into common categories. The homeopath is much more interested in what is distinctive or unique about that individual with ADD rather than those symptoms, such as distractibility and restlessness, which are common to most ADD patients. The homeopath wants to know what the particular child or adult thinks and feels rather than the interpretation of the parent or teacher or therapist.

For example, it is extremely common for children to love pizza and chips. It is much more uncommon if a child raves about artichokes or spinach. We saw a child recently who was fixated on tornadoes and hurricanes. He loved their twirling motion and repeatedly twirled his hands to mimic this motion. This is unusual. Many children like to spend their money on candy and video games. We know of a girl who saved all of her allowance money to send to an organization attempting to save the whales. This is out of the ordinary in our society. It is the odd or quirky symptoms that are much more likely to lead the homeopath to the best medicine for an individual than the normal or common symptoms. It is generally gratifying to the parent and patient to find a health professional whose goal is to spend as much time as necessary to really try to walk a mile in the patient's shoes.

Perceiving the State of Each Person

Each individual has a *state.* That state is the mental-emotional-physical stance that the person has adopted. Take Jimmy, for example, whose story we told in the introduction to this book. Jimmy had been subjected to profound neglect and abuse. His mother had chased him into the bathroom to beat him. Jimmy's response was to keep moving. He moved all the time, even when it was inappropriate or when he needed to sleep. He did anything he could to keep himself busy. Jimmy's hands, legs, mouth, and mind all moved incessantly. This is a state. Perhaps he kept in constant motion out of a subconscious effort to dull his pain or to escape. Whatever the reason, he was in a state of perpetual motion.

Another child in the same situation might respond by closing himself in his room with his books in an effort to hide from the world. Still another might cover up his pain by becoming the class clown and putting on an air of silliness.

The state of a person may have been adopted during a time of past danger or fear. Even when the person is in a very safe environment, the perception of danger may persist. The person may be frozen in that state which served a purpose for coping in the past. Now that state is unnecessary, but it is familiar and may persist for years, decades, or a lifetime. This is particularly true for women who have been subjected to sexual abuse. For years they may remain terrified, or believe sex is painful, or that they do not deserve a loving sexual relationship.

In addition to each person having a unique state, each homeopathic medicine also corresponds to a state. Some medicines have states of terror, others of torment, and still others of an inability to think, concentrate, and remember. There are homeopathic medicines for people who feel pursued and for those whose state is a total lack of confidence. For every imaginable state, there corresponds one homeopathic medicine that best matches that state.

Once that specific medicine is prescribed, an often profound shift can occur. You will read about these shifts throughout this book. It is even possible to shift a state that has been in place for decades. The state of a child or an adult with ADD sometimes shifts quickly and dramatically. It is important to remember that every single person has one state or another. It does not make someone bad or unlovable. People with ADD may irritate others by their excessive interrupting, intrusiveness, and their hyperexcitability. It is usually no fun for the person himself to be this way because of the negative reactions he causes. Most states, however irritating or extreme, can be brought into balance by homeopathic treatment.

Animal, Plant, and Mineral Types

One fascinating model that has emerged in recent years in homeopathy, introduced by Dr. Rajan Sankaran of

Bombay, India, in *The Substance of Homeopathy,* is the concept of animal, plant, and mineral personality types. We think this model will help you begin to grasp the uniqueness of different people that the homeopath endeavors to perceive. Since homeopathic medicines come from the natural world, they can be categorized into the kingdoms of nature: animal, plant, and mineral. People who need medicines made from animal sources will have different characteristics and symptoms from people needing medicines from plant or mineral sources. Once the kingdom is determined, the homeopath must still select the appropriate medicine from that kingdom. This takes considerable experience, so you can understand why it is important to seek treatment from an experienced professional rather than do your own guesswork.

Let's begin with the animal kingdom. Think of animals, from protozoa to elephants. How do they act and what issues seem important to them? Animals move around looking for food, water, sex, a comfortable place to sleep, warmth, and protection from the elements. Wild animals are highly competitive, which is necessary for their survival. They compete for food, mates, territory, and superiority. Animals draw attention to themselves. They often try to be more attractive and colorful than those around them, although some animals are masters of camouflage.

People who need homeopathic medicines from animal sources are animated, expressive, and full of life. They, like animals, are alert and quick to act and react. They often dress attractively and enjoy calling attention to themselves. Their eyes are often striking. These individuals tend to be aggressive, pushy, and competitive and may attack if provoked. They may have issues of jealousy, envy, and competition for work or social position. There are often issues of fighting and such animal-like behaviors as hitting, kicking, biting, scratching, and even growling. These individuals often recount feelings and situations of domination or being dominated. They may have feelings of inferiority and worthlessness. Animals fear loss of power, mates, and territory, and dread isolation, neglect, and rejection. People needing animal remedies may complain of ravenous, or canine, hunger and may tend toward crude, even primitive, behaviors. In general, they have problems getting along with others in their daily lives.

Individuals needing medicines from plant sources think and behave very differently. Plants tend to be sensitive and so are plant-like people. Plants need regular water and sunshine and healthy soil in order to survive. There are, of course, some extremely hardy plants, but most need certain conditions to thrive. Plants try to adapt to weather changes. Plant-like people are much more adaptable than animal types. They often try to go along with others' wishes at the expense of their own needs. They are often soft, gentle people who love nature, plants, and flowers. They very often wear clothing with flower or plant designs. They may lack firm structure and have a changeable nature. Their feelings are often easily hurt.

Just as plants can send out runners to occupy the surrounding space, absorbing what is necessary for life, plant-like people are often diffuse by nature, wandering in thought, speech, and action. They tend to be very emotional. They seek support and nurturing. They are often creative and artistic, and desire to surround themselves with beauty, art, and music. During the homeopathic interview, patients needing plant remedies often wander from subject to subject. They may seem disorganized or whimsical.

Now think of the mineral kingdom. What are minerals like? They are fixed, solid, and structured. People needing mineral remedies tend to have these traits. They are highly organized, orderly, structured individuals. They are concerned with issues of safety, security, performance, finances, or relationships. They are deliberate, determined, and are logical rather than intuitive. They often speak in facts and figures, percentages, and chronological order.

Mineral types tend to choose careers as accountants, engineers, bookkeepers, scientists, computer programmers, and time-management consultants. They place a high emphasis on getting their jobs done efficiently and correctly. They tend to see things in black and white and may become very frustrated with their intuitive, plant-like associates and spouses.

These people like rocks and gems. Their clothing is unusually simple, earth-toned, and often with geometric designs. They often come into the homeopathic interview with a detailed list of symptoms that they have prepared on their computer. Mineral-type individuals may complain of structural problems in their bodies or their lives. They may have difficulties with the minerals in the body resulting in such conditions as bone and teeth problems or muscular cramping.

This animal, plant, and mineral classification is just one example of the many ways a homeopath tries to understand his patients as individuals and find a corresponding homeopathic medicine. You may say that we still use categories, but we do so only to match the person to the medicine. As we listen to each patient, we make every effort to perceive him as a unique individual.

10

——⟨∞⟩——

Understanding and Treating
the Whole Person
An Introduction to
Homeopathic Treatment

The Homeopathic Interview

The core of homeopathic treatment is the homeopathic interview. Each patient is carefully interviewed to discover the individual pattern of symptoms that determines which homeopathic medicine will provide the best treatment. The interview is conducted in a particular way, which enables the homeopath to gather information both by observation and by questioning.

The interview is designed to allow the patient to simply tell her story, including her chief complaint, physical symptoms, mental symptoms, and emotional state. At first the homeopath lets the patient express herself as much as she likes without asking any questions, except perhaps a general opening question such as "What can I help you with?" or "Tell me about yourself."

Listening and observation are the main tasks of the homeopath during the interview. More is to be gained by the homeopath through watching, listening, and waiting than by speaking too much or too soon. From the moment of meeting the patient to the time she checks out at the desk, the homeopath is always looking for clues to the patient's state of mind and body. A great deal can be revealed by a person's body posture, facial expressions, overall demeanor, and degree of animation. The homeopath asks herself, "What kind of person is sitting in front of me? How is she unique? What are her unique symptoms?"

A child with ADD may not be able to sit in one place for even a few minutes of the sixty- to ninety-minute interview. He may wander about the room aimlessly, handling objects, opening drawers, tapping and poking, making noises, and looking for anything to distract himself while generally trashing the office. Toys are played with for a few moments, then broken or discarded for the next object of interest. Running, jumping, hiding under the table, pounding on things, throwing anything not nailed down, and taking things apart are all part of the process. In the meantime, the parent and homeopath will try to share a few bits of information punctuated by scoldings, warnings, and endless explanations about everything in the office and how soon the child can go home. We heard one expert on ADD remark that many children with ADD act like calm little angels when their parents take them to the doctor. This is not often our experience. In an hour-long homeopathic interview, the child often reveals himself clearly. In cases where this is not true, the homeopath relies more heavily on the information provided by parents and teachers.

Even the ADD adult may become easily bored or distracted during the interview process. He will wander from subject to subject and rock, fidget, tap on things, or even pace restlessly while telling his story. The adult with ADD usually has more patience than a child but his attention span can still be quite short. It is frustrating for both the patient and the homeopath to try to follow this rambling, disconnected story with many people, places, and events presented somewhat randomly or in a confused way. When the interview goes like this it may corroborate the diagnosis of ADD, of which the patient may or may not be aware.

Questions are asked to cover any areas of the patient's life or symptoms that are not spontaneously expressed or are of particular interest to the homeopath. Some questions cover general topics such as the person's energy level and sleep, hunger, and thirst patterns, looking for unusual or striking symptoms. One person may only be able to sleep on her right side, with lots of blankets and the window open. Another person will want to sleep in the nude with only a thin sheet and stick his feet out of the bed. One man may have total loss of appetite, while another is ravenous. A women may have insatiable desire for sex or could not care less for it. One patient may have a strong thirst for ice water, while another may only like occasional sips of warm tea. These distinctions help the homeopath find a prescription for the patient.

The particular foods or tastes which the person craves, like coffee, sweets, chocolate, vinegar, spicy foods, and fruit, may lead the homeopath to consider particular homeopathic medicines that are known to relate to certain kinds of cravings. People who need the homeopathic medicine *Nux vomica,* for example, crave spicy food, animal fat, and stimulants, while those requiring *Veratrum album* often desire pickles, sour fruits like lemons, and ice to chew.

The mental and emotional state of the patient is very carefully drawn out and examined by the homeopath. Many patients may think it is like a therapy session, but the intent is to understand thoughts and feelings in order to choose the medicine that can help restore balance to the whole person. Traumatic experiences such as physical and sexual abuse, life-changing events like war, disaster, and famine, formative aspects of childhood, griefs, disappointments, embarrassment and shame, relationship issues, and triumphs and joys are all discussed to explore the feelings and thought patterns that they may have created. Anything in the person's life that has created a lasting effect may be important. Fears, anxieties, and phobias; obsessions, compulsions, and unusual habits; delusions, hallucinations, and peculiar ways of thinking can all be important parts of the mental and emotional state of the patient. The capacity for attention, abstract thought, memory, and concentration are also quite important in characterizing the mental state. These can play a large role in cases of ADD.

The pains, limitations, disabilities, quirks, imbalances, and emotional and mental states of the patient are all regarded as important threads of information, which the homeopath weaves into a picture of unique symptoms of the patient. The patient's state is matched carefully to all the symptom pictures of homeopathic medicines which might be similar, much as the pieces of a jigsaw puzzle are carefully put together to reveal a strikingly beautiful mountain. The homeopath who solves the puzzle not only discovers that the picture is of a mountain, but clearly differentiates between the shape of Mount Rainier and Mount Kilimanjaro. When a very close or exact match is found between the symptoms of the patient and a particular homeopathic medicine, the homeopath can give the medicine with confidence, expecting improvement in the patient's condition.

The Course of Homeopathic Treatment

After the initial visit or phone consultation, you will be asked to have another appointment in five to eight weeks. At that time your progress will be evaluated. If you or your child is responding well to the homeopathic treatment, your homeopath will likely advise you to continue your current treatment program. If you have not responded well or have had only a partial response to the medicine, your homeopath may change the prescription. As your health improves with homeopathic treatment, consultations generally become less frequent. Even when you or your child is doing well, however, your homeopath may want to see you two to four times a year to make sure you are doing as well as possible.

11

---⌐∞⌐---

The Choice Is Yours
What Parents Say About Homeopathic Treatment of ADD and Other Behavioral and Learning Problems

We asked the parents of some of our patients to give us their candid impressions of how they feel that homeopathy has affected their children. We believe that it is very important to give patients and parents of patients a chance to voice their opinions.

"Michael's Behavior Improved Dramatically"

"We did not want to put Michael on drugs. I was very open-minded and willing to try anything except a personality-altering drug. We racked our brains for weeks, knowing there had to be something else out there to help us. Not a drug. That's when we found you and homeopathy. After one appointment with you and a dose of homeopathic medicine, the teachers and counselors were calling me at home to find out what I had done with Michael. His behavior improved dramatically. His schoolwork turned around 180 degrees. He was able to listen and to process information. All this without Ritalin. The teachers changed their mind about Michael's diagnosis of ADD. Any doubts or worries that I had about trying homeopathy for the first time dissipated after the calls from Michael's teacher. Homeopathic medicine has worked wonders with him. I'm thrilled to know that there is an alternative to the traditional pop-a-pill method. Michael's success has even convinced my husband, who is studying to be a paramedic, that there may be a better way."

"Benjie Was Always Wild"

"Benjie had always been really wild and different from the other boys. He was aggressive. He could not sit still and would not respond to adults or to anyone in authority. He was diagnosed with ADD by teachers, our family doctor, and other professionals. When we brought him to see you, you agreed with the diagnosis. After a very thorough interview, you gave him a homeopathic medicine. Almost immediately after taking the medicine, Benjie changed. He calmed down, sat still, and would actually listen. I encourage anyone to get homeopathic help for ADD."

"Homeopathy Has Changed Phil's Whole Attitude . . . and Ours"

"Homeopathic treatment has really made a difference in our home life and in my relationship with Phil. It's so much better. He had somehow gotten the impression from us that there was something wrong with him. Homeopathy has changed his whole attitude and ours. It is so much more relaxed around our house now. Phil can settle down. He can get through the basics of the day without negotiating every little thing. He doesn't scream anymore. I no longer worry about him at school or in new situations. I don't pick him up from school with a sick stomach every day wondering what the teacher will tell me. A close family friend asked me what I had done to help Phil so much. She was amazed."

"I Got My Son Back Again!"

"After our family vacation to Disneyland, I felt like I didn't know Jason anymore. It was as if someone had replaced my child with someone else. He suddenly became hateful and spit and hit. He even spit in his dad's face. Out of nowhere he was disrespectful and could not be satisfied. The only explanation that I can think of is that I was holding his baby sister in my lap during the trip. He started telling us that there was 'a guy in his room.' He was really afraid, which was totally uncharacteristic of him before the trip. Everyone told me it might be because he was sexually abused, but I knew that wasn't the case.

"I was very scared and nervous about the change in his personality. He went from being sweet to very fearful. His fears went away with homeopathic treatment. I felt like I got Jason back again. I think about it often when I look at him. I feel that I lost him temporarily and got him back. Homeopathy is so simple and safe."

"Reese's Ability to Focus Is Remarkably Better Since Homeopathy"

"I was amazed when my son told me that he couldn't concentrate at school because of the constant pictures that went through his head. They only lasted a few seconds each and ranged from pleasant scenarios to scary monsters. He told me they were almost always there. Within days of taking his homeopathic medicine, they started to go away. Two weeks later they were totally gone and have not returned. The length of time that he was able to stay focused at school started increasing and is remarkably better now than it was a year ago."

A Case Where Homeopathy Was Not Helpful

"We turned to homeopathy with our regular doctor's blessings. He had run out of answers for Rich. We tried many different homeopathic medicines over two years. We were dealing with angry, defiant behavior, hyperactivity, inability to focus, and physical tics including throat clearing and spitting. We found some medicines that did wonders with the angry, defiant behavior and hyperactivity or the focus, but the tics were still a problem. Or we found something that helped the tics, but not his other behaviors. Due to the severity of his symptoms and how profoundly they affected his daily life, especially in junior high school, we finally took him to a Tourette's syndrome research specialist in California. He is now on a combination of drugs and is doing considerably better. I still believe that if Rich had more time and less pressing circumstances in his life, his homeopathic doctor could have found a medicine to meet his needs. She certainly found one for me that changed my life for the better and helped me cope with being a mother living with a child with ADHD and Tourette's syndrome."

"Before Homeopathy He Drew Sharks. Now He Draws Funny Cartoon Characters"

"Jay is introverted and shy by nature, yet can play very cooperatively with other children. He can become angry quickly with verbal outbursts. After his little sister was born he developed recurring impetigo. He fell into the position of a silent middle child. When he was excluded by the other children at school, he told us he felt terrible and wanted to kill himself. He repeated this despairing statement on four separate occasions. He began to draw unsuspecting swimmers being devoured by ferocious sharks.

"After being treated homeopathically, Jay's sweet personality returned. His impetigo cleared up. He acted more kindly to his sister and became cooperative again. He stopped drawing sharks and began drawing cartoons or comical figures. He went to a new school where he made many friends and was elected class president. Recently he remarked, 'I don't let it bother me anymore when people put me down. I just go on with what I'm doing. It doesn't hurt my feelings like it did before.' "

"He's Not in Special Help Classes Anymore"

"Ray has come a long way since beginning homeopathy. He had lots of learning problems in the past which, over time, affected his self-esteem. Ray is now doing much better at school. His grades in English have come up from D's and F's to B's. He no longer attends special help classes. He is very happy about that and so are we."

"Allie Hasn't Had a Problem with Ear Infections Since We Saw You and She's Much More Cooperative"

"I think you already know that I think homeopathy is wonderful. I first came to you with both of the girls two and a half years ago. Allie had ear infections which her pediatrician had treated with many different courses of antibiotics. I didn't want to keep doing that so I brought her to see you. You worked with us. We found a homeopathic medicine for her and her ear infections cleared up. She hasn't had a problem with them since. I remember that she was two years old when we first saw you and she always had a fear of dogs. Ever since that first medicine you gave her, I haven't been able to keep her away from them. Every time she sees a dog now, she asks about it. It's amazing.

"As far as disposition, Allie has been a challenge. When she has had bouts of being difficult to get along with and uncooperative, fussy, clingy, and doesn't want to do what she's asked, you've given her medicines that have really helped. She's become more receptive and open and cooperative and much more enjoyable to associate with. She also had a bad, recurrent cough which you have been successful in treating.

"Allie's sister, Bri, didn't have as many problems, but when I first brought her to see you she was always picking her nose, scratching her bottom, grinding her teeth at night, and couldn't wait for anything. You gave her a medicine that cleared up all of those symptoms."

Feedback from a Relieved Teacher

"Luis' transformation after taking his first dose of homeopathic medicine was as immediate as I could have ever imagined. He went from being very unfocused to being an active member of his class. Instead of being aggressive, he became aware of and open to learning appropriately. He got very involved in classroom projects, especially those with insects, bugs, butterflies, and worms. In fact, he became a real leader in the class. It was a night-and-day kind of change. It made all the difference in my work with him. Doors opened for Luis that were closed to him before. I give homeopathy my raves and raves and raves. I appreciate 100 percent the changes in Luis. I had so much trouble with him before he started homeopathy that I was seriously thinking of quitting my job!"

12

Chunk Down to Keep Up

Coping Strategies for People with ADD

You Are Not Your ADD

Remember that you are a unique, worthwhile, one-of-a-kind human being. You are yourself, not a label or a diagnosis. You may have behaviors, characteristics, and tendencies that annoy, provoke, and push away your family, teachers, and friends. But those are only your behaviors, not the real you. Regardless of how long you have been diagnosed with ADD, how it affects your relationship with others, and whether or not you are on medications, it is important that you and others remember who you really are. Many people diagnosed with ADD may be very bright and extremely creative. Find avenues to express your creativity and discover those activities that you really love.

Understimulate Rather than Overstimulate

People of any age with a tendency to be restless and distracted tend to be more susceptible than the average person to stimulants of all kinds. This includes caffeine, whether in coffee, tea, or pop; extended periods of time in front of the computer or television; loud music with a fast beat; excessive amounts of sugar, or any sugar on an empty stomach; recreational drugs; fluorescent lights; and high-speed, high-stress, high-anxiety situations. It is not that you need to avoid these substances or influences all the time or forever. Just be aware that they will tend to make you more wired and edgy.

Balance your exposure to stimulation with calming activities such as walking out in nature, listening to relaxing music in a dimly lit or dark room, drinking soothing herb teas such as chamomile and peppermint, and eating more natural foods that are whole grains and protein rather than junk foods high in sugar. If you are feeling nervous or having trouble falling asleep, stretch your body and take a few deep breaths. It is amazing how much a few minutes of slow, deep breathing can change how you feel and calm you down.

Chunk Down

No, chunking down does not mean eating a bar of candy. It means taking one step at a time. If you have three pages of math homework, for example, just sit down and get started. Do one problem at a time. If you get stuck, make a note so that you can go back to it later, then go on. Do not let yourself get up to do something else until you finish. Then, when you have done all that you can, ask for help if you need it. When you finish your whole assignment, give yourself a reward. This is called positive reinforcement.

Once your subconscious mind knows that you will be rewarded when you complete a task, it will have much more of an incentive to push you forward. If there are areas where you become continually stuck, tell someone about them so that you can address them in a positive, direct way.

Everything in Its Place

Develop a system of organization and follow it. It does not matter what that system is as long as it works for you. It may be a notebook or a set of file folders or a book bag that has a place for pens and pencils. You may want to ask a very organized person to help you set up your system.

Once you have your system, develop a routine. When you go to class or work and are given an assignment, have a particular place where you write it down and put it away. Keep your book bag in the same place every day, whether it is a locker or in your desk. Take it home every night, along with any additional items that you might need.

One of the biggest challenges for people diagnosed with ADD is to remember what they are supposed to do and where they put things. The more organized a system they can create for themselves, the easier it is for them to keep it all together.

Keep a Schedule

The best way to get everything done that you need to is to keep a consistent schedule. It may sound boring, but it is a great way to keep on track. Ask your parents or spouse to remind you if you get off schedule.

If you get up at the same time every morning, leave the house at the same time, and have a schedule for your homework or other activities, you will get into a groove. The more you change your schedule, the easier it is for you to forget what you need to do or where you were about to go.

Write It Down!

Whether you are eight or eighty, get in the habit of making lists to aid your memory. If you think of something that you need to do, write it down: what, when, where, a phone number, or any other relevant information. Keep a little notebook with you all the time in a place that you will remember. The greatest list in the world is useless if you cannot find it.

Be Silent Now and Then

A little silence can do wonders for a busy mind. When you catch yourself between tasks or appointments, force yourself to sit down for a few minutes to take a break. Rather than immediately clicking on the television and channel surfing, an activity guaranteed to overstimulate your mind, just be quiet for a few minutes. Listen to the sounds around you. Give yourself an opportunity each day to do absolutely nothing, even if it is just for a few moments. This attitude of silence can become a habit. Gradually, day by day, month by month, you will become calmer and your nervous system will feel more relaxed.

Burn Off Some Ya Yas Through Exercise

A great deal of nervous energy can be released through vigorous exercise. Pounding a softball with your bat or zipping around the block on your bike can be very rejuvenating. Vigorous exercise gets the diaphragm moving and the endorphins flowing. If you feel about to jump out of your skin or on the verge of screaming, exercise. Choose a form of exercise that you enjoy to increase your likelihood of doing it regularly. Remember to breathe while you exercise and to take your time. If you are a nervous, restless person, it is best to choose a type of exercise that is not speed-driven and competitive.

Know Your Limits

When you begin to feel that you are reaching your limit of stress, stop! Don't push yourself further for the moment. Take a couple of deep breaths or walk around, whichever is appropriate. You may want to tell whomever you are with that you need to take a short break. Ask yourself what you need at that moment to feel calm and relaxed and then do it. If you feel your mind or your heart start to race, realize that you are getting nervous. When we become stressed, our sympathetic nervous system and fight-or-flight mechanisms kick in. Stop and let your parasympathetic mechanisms take over so that you will feel more relaxed.

13

—⁓∞⁓—

The Ups and Downs of Living with an ADD Child
Tips for Parents

Enhancing Homeopathic Treatment

In our practice we have seen homeopathy stimulate tremendous positive change in children with ADD. In order for this change to become permanent, it is important for your child to feel loved, supported, and directed at home. Here are some behavioral and attitudinal suggestions that can help you support your child's healing process.

Appreciate the Uniqueness of Your Child

Many of the children with ADD and related problems whom we have treated are fascinating, engaging, charming, intensely curious, and brilliant. They may also drive everyone around them crazy. Conventional medicine attempts to categorize people in order to treat them. This en masse approach does not recognize the precious individuality that makes each of us unique.

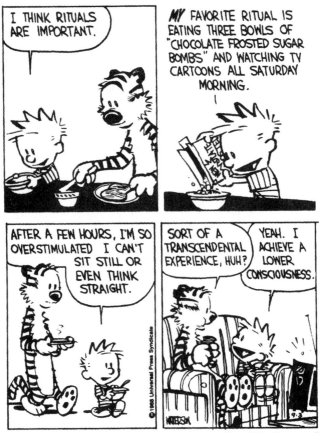

Calvin and Hobbes © (1988) Watterson. Distributed by Universal Press Syndicate. Reprinted with permission. All rights reserved.

Even the most negative and challenging children have their endearing traits and moments.

Remember that your child is one of a kind (even if there are moments when you wonder if he's the wrong kind!). He may not meet any of your expectations. If so, let him be himself. A friend of ours who is the mother of a child with ADD shared some advice that has often helped her over the years. It was advice given by a physician to parents of developmentally impaired children, but she felt it was very apt for parents of children with ADD. He counseled, "Imagine that you are planning a wonderful trip to Italy. You get out a map of Italy and plan to go to Florence and Siena and Rome. You take some classes in Italian. Your mouth is watering at the mere thought of freshly made pasta. You pack your bags, get on the plane, and are off to Italy. The plane lands. You look around, bewildered, and realize that you are in Holland, not Italy. Initially you are very disappointed. Then you think about the tulips and the Rembrandts and the windmills and begin to enjoy yourself. You realize that the country is very different. It's not what you expected, but it's still a wonderful place." That story stuck in our friend's mind and helped her through the many challenging moments of raising a child with ADD.

Many of our adult patients' biggest emotional problems result from their parents' unmet expectations which they are forever trying to live up to long after their parents are even on this earth. You may have been a Fulbright scholar and your daughter may be two grades behind in her reading. Or perhaps you were a college football star and your son is too timid even to try out for the team. But maybe that same child loves animals and dreams of setting up a wild animal shelter. Or maybe he is fascinated with tornadoes and hurricanes, like one of our patients, and will grow up to be a fantastic meteorologist. You never know. What is most important is that he grows up to be himself.

Don't Blame Yourself or Your Child

We are all trying to do the best we can at any time. Whether you or your child's ADD is connected to genes, abuse or neglect, or naive parenting skills, there is no point in obsessing over blame. Learn as much as you can to help yourself or your child and take whatever concrete steps seem best to fit you and your family's situation and needs. Adults and children with ADD usually mean well. They are not trying to be obnoxious, terminally restless, and unbearable to be around. They generally want to be accepted and liked, to learn and fit in. But the more their behaviors alienate them from their family, teachers, and peers, the worse they feel about themselves. Their self-esteem plummets and there is often considerable self-reproach or even self-hatred, whether or not it is obvious to others around. Most children with ADD already know they are screwing up. Reminding them of their every mistake only serves to make them feel even more terrible about what they often cannot consciously control.

The ability of people to change their behaviors after they are positively reinforced is no myth. Whenever you can catch your child doing something good, immediately praise him. Let him know that you really appreciate it when he does something well. Children who are always criticized will live up, or rather down, to their parents poor expectations of them. If you are convinced that your child is dumb or that he will never listen to you, he will probably prove you right. People with ADD need clear limits, routines, and instructions, but nobody needs blame.

One Step at a Time and Keep It Simple

Children with ADD generally have problems following directions, particularly if they are given all at once in a series. Keep instructions and expectations simple, one step at a time. These children are not known for their ability to multi-task but are often quite capable of completing tasks successfully if they clearly understand what is expected of them. By asking your child to do one thing at a time, the likelihood of success is much greater, your child will feel better about his ability to handle demands, and you can positively reinforce each job well done. Once he is capable of simple tasks like making his bed or feeding the dog or taking out the trash, then you can develop more sophisticated strategies, such as chore check-off lists or schedules.

Predictable Routines

Maria Montessori, in her study of children, found that children feel most comfortable and function best with order and routine. This is especially true of children who are distractible and unfocused. A schedule that remains the same day after day may seem boring and rote, but is very helpful for children with ADD. Knowing what they are expected to do, and when and where they need to be helps considerably to cut down on being at loose ends and bouncing off the walls. These children need clear guidance and direction, and, most of all, consistency. Whether they attend school or are home-schooled, knowing where they are going day after day will add a helpful organization to their minds and lives.

Set Limits and Be Consistent

These children often push boundaries and have problems with defiance, impulsivity, and feeling out of control in many areas of their lives. Although an excessively rigid environment can make them even more rebellious and defiant, clear, loving limits are essential. Let your child know clearly what is expected of her and what the consequence will be if the expectation is not met. Time-outs, restrictions, household chores, and family commitments do not have to be punitive. They can be a means of establishing firm and reasonable guidelines. It is important that the guidelines, expectations, and consequences be followed consistently by both parents. This is especially important if the parents are divorced and two households, and sometimes four parents, are involved.

One-on-One

People with ADD often find communication much easier if it is limited to one other person. The more stimulation, conversation, and input, the more potential for distraction and confusion. Some children with ADD are so sensitive and distractible that the slightest noise will disrupt their focus. We treated one little girl whose attention was inevitably diverted every time the cat walked by. She just had to run over and pet and tease it until both little girl and feline were overwhelmed. After homeopathy, her concentration improved considerably and the cat was not a constant distraction. Siblings or peers can be even more attention-grabbing, much less an entire classroom. This is particularly true when more than one child in the family has characteristics of ADD. Consider spending regular time one-on-one with your ADD child. This can be a meal, an outing, a movie, or a walk. It offers a time where the child can have less input and develop better communication skills.

Choose Nonstimulating Activities

Have you ever sat at the computer for four hours straight working on a project or playing computer games? For children who are already over-amped, this can have an intensely mind-jangling effect. The same is true of long periods spent watching television. Try to help your child find activities that actually calm the nervous system such as taking a walk together in nature, particularly where there are trees and water, both of which have a calming effect on the mind. Participate together in recreational activities that burn energy but do not overstimulate. Swimming, tennis, ice skating, yoga or stretching, tai chi, and aikido are much more soothing than aerobic dance, sprinting, and other noisy, fast activities. Many children with ADD feel awkward and uncoordinated. Helping them to find a sport or activity in which they can succeed is a great way not only to calm a strung-out nervous system, but to enhance self-esteem.

Become a Master of Communication with Your Child

Learn what it takes to communicate well with your child. One of the best techniques is called *active listening* and comes from the *Parent Effectiveness Training* method of Thomas Gordon, M.Ed. A major problem with many ADD children is that they selectively tune out. They often hear only part of what is said to them. Even if they hear every single word, they often do not acknowledge having taken in the information, so you feel unheard. Developing successful communication strategies will not only greatly enhance enjoyable conversation with your child, but will also provide a model of how she can communicate well with other children. This is particularly important for the type of child with ADD who feels very self-conscious about her inability to express herself and then clams up in the classroom or social settings and ends up feeling isolated.

Cultivate Your Sense of Humor

Having an ADD child can push your buttons, make you want to scream, and drive you crazy. These children are also often very funny. We are not suggesting that you roll over laughing when your little angel puts your watch in the microwave or pours cement down your kitchen sink. It is obviously not helpful to positively reinforce destructive tendencies. But there are moments when you can become a child again yourself, act just as mischievous as he does, and just play together. Some children may act so foolishly and silly that you do not want to further encourage their inappropriate behaviors. But no matter how much your child's behaviors upset you, remember to find ways to laugh and have fun together. ADD children's lives can be filled with many moments of hyperintensity. They need opportunities to lighten up as much as you do.

Don't Let the ADD Destroy Your Happiness, Sanity, and Marriage

Watch for the red flags that indicate that you are depressed, stuffing rage, or have sunk into a state of apathy about your family and your life. Loving and raising an ADD child has its many challenges, but do not forget about the rest of your life. This may mean diligently seeking out babysitters or after-school or weekend activities for your child so that you can sometimes get a break. As a parent, you need to find ways to cultivate your own peace, happiness, and creativity. It is a big mistake to sublimate your own needs for ten to twenty years while you devote every waking hour to your hyperactive child. Don't lose yourself in the process of raising your family. If the tension generated by your child's behavioral problems creates significant dissention between you and your spouse, partner, or the other children, seek out help in the form of counseling or a support group.

Fight Only the Big Battles

Do whatever you need to do to maintain your equilibrium, be it therapy, going to church, meditating, deep breathing, a support group, or taking a walk. Set clear limits and identify the issues that matter the most. Some children with ADD will make a mountain out of every molehill and need very little to storm into a tantrum or argument. We are not suggesting that you walk on eggshells twenty-four hours a day, but rather that you save your energy for what is really important. You may want your daughter to bathe every morning, brush her teeth twice a day, and wear clean, ironed clothes to school. She may not care less and the cleanliness issue may turn into a war. Maybe you feel very strongly about your child minimizing junk foods, while he is perfectly happy living on cheeseburgers, fries, milkshakes, and cokes. You may have a strong standard about getting all A's, but your child is satisfied with barely passing her classes.

If you have a major battle with your child over every one of these issues, your life at home will be a constant struggle. Consider some compromises. Be clear about those issues on which you stand absolutely firm, but give your kid some slack in other areas. Flexibility and adaptation are necessary qualities in a parent. Remember the story about Italy and Holland. Take some time to admire the tulips even though you were hoping for a romantic dinner of ravioli and Chianti.

Exploring Behavioral Strategies

Many insightful and extremely useful books provide effective guidelines for helping children's behavior, but no single book or approach will work for everyone. We were recently asked by a school nurse whether we routinely recommend behavior modification to the parents of our ADD patients. Stimulants, antidepressants, and other conventional medications for ADD often affect only one area of a child's problems such as concentration or impulsivity.

Homeopathic medicines affect the whole child. Behavior improves along with concentration, attitude, attentiveness, and physical complaints. The child's behavioral problems are generally sufficiently addressed with homeopathy, making extensive behavior modification unnecessary. In cases where some behavioral interventions are helpful, however, by all means use them.

Get Treatment for Your Own ADD If You Have It

We have found that many children with ADD have parents with ADD. The traits may have been merely a mild annoyance in school and no longer are an interference in daily life. In other cases, however, the parent has such strong tendencies toward distractibility, hurriedness, forgetfulness, and inability to keep commitments and to follow through on tasks that the child cannot help but be affected. We treated one woman with two children diagnosed with ADD. She could not remember anything that she had to do unless she wrote it down on two calendars. She even forgot to pick her children up at school. We know other parents who simply cannot remember, time and time again, to call us for their phone appointments for their ADD children. If you have significant ADD yourself, get help. It may be enough to read some books on strategies for coping with adult ADD, or you may find the answer in therapy, a support group, homeopathy, or other alternative or conventional treatment.

Follow Your Intuition Regarding Diagnosis and Treatment

Educate yourself as much as possible regarding diagnosis and treatment alternatives, then follow your gut feeling. What is right for your child's best friend, or even for her older sibling, may not be right for her. Do not let relatives, friends, or other parents convince you to follow a route that does not feel right to you. The path that you follow with your child may have repercussions for many years. The more you can relax and take time to do what you really believe in for your child, the fewer problems you and she are likely to have later.

14

---⸜∞⸝---

A Revved-Up Classroom
For Teachers, Counselors, and School Nurses

Be Open-Minded

Parents have differing belief systems and healthcare orientations. They choose different options in dealing with their children's problems and challenges. No single way is right or wrong. Every parent who conscientiously raises a child wants to help that child be happy and healthy. A parent with a strong belief in conventional medicine will seek the route of medications. A parent with a strong belief in and experience with alternative medicine will likely opt for a more natural route. Regardless of your personal opinion about what that child needs, the choice is up to the parents and child. Be respectful if the parents do not want to give their child drugs until they have explored other options. If they do try homeopathy or other alternative therapies, support them in that process. Realize that any new therapy should be given an adequate time frame, usually four to six months. Then help the parents, objectively, to assess the results of the new treatment.

No Two Children Are Alike

Try to understand that each child is unique. Each child, just like adults, wants to be happy and cooperative. But there are often obstacles. Perhaps that child comes from a long line of closet alcoholics or was sexually abused as an infant or his mother was a crack addict during the pregnancy or she was unduly reprimanded from the time she was an infant for not behaving perfectly. There are countless reasons for why children have behavioral and learning problems. No matter how mean, defiant, or impossible a child is, at some level he wants to be loving and cooperative and, most of all, he needs help. This is sometimes difficult to remember at the end of a long day in a classroom of forty children, but it is important. Try to climb inside each child's mind and body so you can understand and appreciate her unique experience of life.

Your Feedback Is Extremely Important

Homeopaths base a child's prescription on what is most striking or unique about that individual child. Whatever information you can give to the parents about what you find unusual about their child, either in a positive or negative sense, will help the homeopath to select the best medicine. This is true both before the child begins to take the medicine and during the course of treatment. One of the most significant ways that we measure improvement in the case of a child with ADD is to hear how much better he is adjusting to, performing in, relating to, and enjoying his classroom.

How You Can Support the Homeopathic Treatment Process

- Don't pressure parents to medicate their child with Ritalin or other conventional drugs to treat ADD. Let the parents decide.
- Notice how the child is behaving and learning so that you can provide the parents with as much specific feedback as possible.
- Be aware of those few substances and factors which interfere with homeopathic treatment that may be present in the classroom (coffee, eucalyptus, camphor, menthol) and do not encourage the child to use them.
- Talk with parents of children who have been helped by alternative treatment of ADD so that you can be better informed about the available choices.
- Understand that homeopathic medicines have a much longer action than stimulants or antidepressants. Do not be surprised when parents tell you their child receives his homeopathic medication only once a day, once a week, or even only several times a year.

What to Expect in Your Classroom

It can take anywhere from one day to one month after a homeopathic medicine is given before the effects are noticeable. You may notice that the child's behavior is initially worse for a few days or even two weeks. This is more likely to occur if the parents have simultaneously chosen to discontinue the child's stimulants or antidepressant medication. It may take several months, or occasionally longer, to find the homeopathic medicine that is most effective for the individual child.

Once that medicine is found, you can expect to see a significant improvement in the child's attitude, behavior, learning abilities, and other physical and emotional symptoms. The changes may be subtle or dramatic. With the correct homeopathic medicine, you will generally see at least a 50 percent overall improvement in the child, usually more. Sometimes there are occasional periods of relapse, where the initial symptoms return to some extent. If you notice this, be sure to inform the parents.

15

A Meeting of the Conventional and Unconventional Worlds
For Psychologists, Psychiatrists, Pediatricians, and Other Physicians

Back to the Hippocratic Oath

Whether or not you believe in alternative therapies or homeopathy, you probably remember the main tenet of the Hippocratic oath: First do no harm. Homeopathic medicines may cause an initial worsening of symptoms, generally lasting no more than a week, but do not have side effects like conventional medicines. If you knew that a natural substance free of side effects, rather than a stimulant or antidepressant, could help many children and adults with ADD, wouldn't you consider that option for your patients? And what if you personally heard from parents of numerous children whose ADD had been helped for at least a year or more with an alternative therapeutic approach? And what if you attended a clinical case conference, along with over a hundred other physicians, documenting case histories and showing videotapes of patients who responded very positively to a natural approach to ADD? Wouldn't you be interested?

Homeopathic Medicine Is Not a Placebo

You may have heard that homeopathic medicines could not possibly work because they do not contain enough of the original substance to be biochemically active. Or that the only reason they work is because the patient believes in them—a pure placebo effect. Homeopathy admittedly does not work on a biochemical level. Nor does acupuncture. These types of medicine are effective because they are forms of energy medicine. We do not yet fully understand how to measure, analyze, or evaluate energy medicine. But, just as acupuncture has been used very effectively for centuries, homeopathy has also shown considerable clinical success for the past 200 years and is widely accepted in many parts of the world.

How could homeopathy act only as a placebo when it is very clear to the homeopath that the correct homeopathic medicine works and incorrect ones do not? If homeopathy were only a placebo, why would the same patients respond dramatically to one homeopathic medicine and not to another? And why would some patients who do not believe at all in homeopathy still respond very well to treatment and others who have great trust and confidence in their homeopathic practitioner not receive benefit? And why would homeopathy work so effectively with animals and infants?

We ask that you open your minds to the possibility that a therapy exists that is very effective but that we do not fully understand. We invite you to talk to us and to other homeopathic practitioners frankly about our successes and failures. We invite you to our clinical case conferences to judge for yourselves whether homeopathy works. We invite you to talk to our patients who have received benefit from homeopathy so that you know our successes are real.

What About Scientific Research?

The crucible of effectiveness for medical therapies is often considered to be research. "What are the relevant statistics in homeopathic research?" you ask. We ask you to take a look at our section on research in chapter 6. We know that homeopathic research is in its infancy, mostly due to lack of funding. A number of medical doctors in the homeopathic community are engaged in planning research studies and seeking funding for that purpose. The Office of Alternative Medicine, in Bethesda, Maryland, recently awarded a grant for a homeopathic research project on head injuries involving Edward Chapman, a homeopathic physician on the faculty of Harvard University Medical School. Our community is actively involved in promoting more high-quality studies on the clinical effectiveness of homeopathy.

In the meantime, however, we ask you to take a look at the case studies in this book. They are authentic cases from our clinical practice, though the names have been changed to protect confidentiality. Can you honestly say that you are not impressed by the effectiveness of homeopathy with these patients?

Why Not Be Open to a New Paradigm?

We are not asking you to give up your principles and practice of conventional medicine, although if you do want to study homeopathy seriously, there are a number of excellent courses available. What we are asking is that you keep an open mind. Perhaps you are one of those people who were initially skeptical about acupuncture, but have now changed your mind because you have seen it work. We believe you will have the same experience with homeopathy.

We recently spoke with a well-respected child psychiatrist who is outspokenly opposed to the use of stimulants and antidepressants to treat ADD. He told us that to consider homeopathy would be to go too far out on a limb as far as his professional credibility. How, we ask, could he read the cases in this book and not have his interest and curiosity piqued? Aren't we on the same team in our efforts to find safe, effective, and lasting answers to help sufferers of ADD and related problems?

Will Homeopathy Interfere with the Medications that You Prescribe?

The answer is clearly no. Homeopathic medicine in no way diminishes the effectiveness of conventional medicine. As the patient improves under homeopathic treatment, however, she may need to take a lower dose of the conventional medicine in order to achieve the same desired effect. Over time the desired effect can often be achieved without the conventional medicine. But isn't that what you would want for your patient anyway . . . to be healthy and free of prescription medications?

A Dose of Ritalin Lasts for Four Hours. How Can a Dose of Homeopathic Medicine Last for Months or Years?

This is one of the paradoxes of homeopathy. Once the energy system of the body has been brought into balance through the use of a homeopathic medicine, the effect will last until the momentum stops, much like a spinning top eventually ceases to spin. The duration of action depends on a number of factors, including the vitality of the patient, the severity of the symptoms, the patient's environment, stresses, and exposure to specific factors which could potentially interfere with homeopathic treatment. In the case of a child with ADD it is very common for a single dose of a homeopathic medicine to last six months or longer.

Some homeopathic practitioners use lower potencies more often. What is most important in homeopathy is to find the correct medicine for the patient. The frequency and potency of the medicine is a matter of case management.

When Is It Time for a Patient to Give Up on Homeopathy?

It is more accurate to ask when it is time to give up on a particular homeopath. Just as you might suggest that a patient who has worked with one psychiatrist, psychologist, or physician for a period of time and is dissatisfied should consider consulting a different one, we would recommend a change of homeopaths. However, a good rule of thumb is to give an experienced homeopathic physician or practitioner six months to a year before seeking another opinion or deciding that homeopathy is ineffective for that individual.

PART THREE

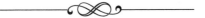

Real Stories of Real People

Successful Homeopathic Treatment of ADD

16

―――⌐◈⌐―――

"Won't I Ever Outgrow This?"
Adults with ADD

Paul Wender, M.D., in his scholarly book *Attention-Deficit Hyperactivity Disorder in Adults,* traces the development of the standard symptoms of ADD from childhood to adulthood.[1] Adults experience persistent, sometimes severe, problems with attention and concentration and may find routine desk jobs impossible or may be labeled as chronic underachievers. They remain distractible, may need frequent reminders when they are given instructions, and often leave tasks uncompleted. These people may seem like they are off in another world and may not hear what is said to them. They frequently forget where they put their possessions and may forget appointments, pay bills late, and appear to be irresponsible, although they might be quite conscientious. Their desks or files are likely to confound any organized person, even though they may actually know where everything is. It is curious that some of these absentminded professor types are extremely brilliant and may be leaders in their fields. They are often inventors,

---

[1] Paul H. Wender, *Attention Deficit Hyperactivity Disorder in Adults* (New York/ Oxford: Oxford University Press, 1995).

scientists, philosophers, and theoreticians—careers where their minds soar and others can pick up the day-to-day pieces of life.

Adults with ADD may be clumsy and awkward. Their social skills may be underdeveloped. The impulsivity of childhood which leads one to jump off a roof or climb a high beam may turn into fast driving, playing the futures market, or any other form of risky behavior. They may exhibit tremendous restlessness, just as they did as children, flitting from one job, task, or idea to the next. As you will see in the following cases, these individuals may fall apart at the seams under stress or overstimulation.

Stuck in High Gear

We are often asked, "Will I grow out of ADD?" The answer is maybe. Many children with traits of hyperactivity, restlessness, distractibility, and impulsivity, if untreated, continue to have these same characteristics throughout their lives. The prevalence of ADD in adults is estimated at 2 to 7 percent of the adult population.[2] We have noticed that some of the children brought to us for ADD are carbon copies of one or both of their parents. The mother often reports, "Billy's dad's the same way. He can't pay attention to save his life. I have to ask him questions six times, just like Billy." Or Billy's mother might report that, although his dad has grown out of his ADD traits, as a child he got in trouble for the exact same things Billy is doing now. Adults who read about ADD often experience a revelation when they read about the subject as they finally understand why they had so many

[2] Ibid., 74.

problems reading, paying attention, and completing tasks. When it comes to ADD, it is never too late to begin homeopathic treatment.

Who Has Time to Sleep?

Carl came to see us at age thirty-seven. Frightened by a strong family history of cancer, he hoped we could strengthen his immune system and increase his chances of avoiding cancer. Carl suffered from congenital hearing loss, also a family trait.

"I tend to work on a crisis basis. I procrastinate and do everything inefficiently. My family is riddled with cancer: my father, mother, and lots of other relatives have had cancer. Preventive medicine doesn't always fit into my lifestyle. I've always had convenient excuses. I like to think of myself as extremely easygoing, but stress affects me. I rebel against others' expectations by procrastinating. Then I feel ashamed when I fall short of their expectations. I berate myself because I'm lazy."

Carl had a history of compulsive drinking and recreational drugs use. A man of excess, once Carl started anything, he just could not quit. He enjoyed engaging in sex as often as possible and masturbated frequently. He had a history of venereal warts as well as herpes on the mouth and canker sores. We noticed that Carl fidgeted incessantly during the interview.

A software programmer, Carl described his concentration as "almost hypnotic in focus" and his memory as extremely good, yet his follow-through was sporadic. It was all or nothing with Carl. He had no clue how to pace himself. When he listened to a song, he felt compelled to play it over and over again. A heavy-duty partier in college, he got into the habit of working all night. He worked regularly up to forty-eight hours straight without sleeping, then napped for six hours to catch up before beginning the cycle again. Carl's perfect schedule was to stay up until 2 or 3 A.M. and sleep until 10 or 11 A.M. the next day. "I've never been a morning person. Only under duress will I get up."

Food was also done to excess. Sour foods and key lime pie were his favorites. The more sour the taste, the better he liked it. As a child, Carl loved taking a jar of lemon juice out of the refrigerator and mixing it with sugar to make a sour paste. He also had a strong desire for Granny Smith apples, really tart and crisp, as well as salty foods and buttermilk. Carbonated soft drinks were Carl's beverage of choice.

Recurrent sinus problems and hay fever bugged Carl. A serious teeth grinder, he wondered if this habit might be a reflection of anger that he held within instead of expressing it to those who expected things of him. Carl was fearless. He enjoyed taking chances and doing things other people might perceive as risky.

We gave Carl a homeopathic nosode called *Medorrhinum*. What was most unusual about him was his intensity in everything he did. Driven to do everything to excess, there was no middle of the road for Carl. His gears were all the way on or all the way off. We also prescribed this medicine for him because of his restless, erratic temperament. Carl had an intensity that was striking, even after we talked with him for just a few minutes. Life for Carl was a world of one intense experience after another. People needing this medicine often have very poor follow-through as Carl described. They may have severe memory problems, though Carl did not, as well as a compulsive bent, history of warts, and a strong desire for sour foods and salt.

At his first return visit six weeks later, Carl reported that he felt moodier and more short-tempered for the first two days following the homeopathic treatment, then noticed an increase in his dandruff and teeth clenching for two weeks. He then found himself waking at six in the morning regardless of when he went to sleep. He experienced a burst of productivity and had accomplished a great deal.

Two months later, Carl reported that his mind was clear and fast. He was not procrastinating as much. He no longer waited until the last minute to write papers. He was engaged in more long-range planning. He was no longer staying up as late. He was in bed now by 1 A.M. instead of 2 or 3. His warts disappeared completely. He

Medorrhinum (nosode)

People like Carl are very hurried mentally, their minds crowded with a thousand thoughts at once. They love to stay up late and as children can be very difficult to put to bed, causing them also to be difficult to wake up the next morning. People who need this medicine often like to sleep on their stomachs or in the knee-chest position. They crave extremes of experience and are very passionate, wanting to do everything to the max. They may be sexually precocious with a tendency to masturbate. Mentally they may seem dull or too intense. They are forgetful and easily distracted. Cruel or loving to animals, they are also sensitive to nature. They fear the dark and monsters. They bite their fingernails or toenails. Diaper rash, sinusitis, warts, asthma, and arthritis are typical physical problems. People needing *Medorrhinum* often love oranges, unripe fruit, ice, sweets, salt, and fat.

had a new girlfriend with whom he had a very active sexual relationship and he no longer felt the urge to masturbate.

Homeopathic treatment continued to help Carl, except when he resorted to recreational drugs, which interfered with the treatment. Over the two and one-half years of treatment, homeopathy helped him to channel his energy in more positive directions. He became more able to deal with others' expectations openly and honestly. He stopped pretending he had done something which he had not, which had gotten him into lots of trouble before. His excessive tendencies diminished and he finally found a moderate pace for himself.

"I Feel Like I'm Jumping Out of My Skin"

At age twenty-five, superachiever Jill sought out homeopathic care due to "nervous symptoms." She had always felt nervous. It was an internal feeling that others often did not notice. "There's an awful lot that I can't get done. I become tense. I can feel like I'm gonna jump right out of my skin. I get hot. If feels like a hot flash, an adrenaline rush. I feel weak in the knees. When I become nervous, I feel a sloshy, gurgling sensation in my abdomen and get diarrhea. I was diagnosed with colitis three years ago, but I had the beginnings of an ulcer at nineteen."

Jill felt jumpy about her family and about keeping up with life. She had raised her young son as a single mom while taking a full-credit load at the university and graduated Phi Beta Kappa cum laude with a degree in physical therapy. She was a highly responsible person, always thinking of what she needed to do. Hurried inside, she often became so nervous that she hyperventilated.

At those times, her fingers turned blue. It was hard for Jill to relax unless she was exhausted or sick. She remembered enjoying having the flu as a child so she could relax. She had always been a worry wart. At her third birthday party, she remembered that her birthday wish was that the stock market would go up because she was worried about the family finances. Jill's nickname as a child was "Chatterbox." Her mother trained her not to bother people. It was hard for Jill to keep her hands off of the other girls' curly hair and to avoid touching things in stores.

She complained of a heightened sensitivity to her environment. Jill felt oversensitive to music, weather, and to feelings inside a room. Not much escaped her. She had an exaggerated startle response and reflexes. It was as if she were always ready to explode. She became so angry at times that it scared her. She used to be a heavier drinker. Once when drunk she tried to choke her ex-husband.

Jill was constantly "fighting against a busy depression." "I have to stay busy. I'm not good at home unbusy. I'd like to feel more comfortable with myself doing nothing. I have the urge to touch people, arm wrestle, put my hands on their heads, but I hold myself back because of social rules. I think about it all the time. I have impulses to kiss people I don't know, but I don't allow myself to act on them. I rarely meet a couple that I don't imagine in bed together. My mind is full of socially unacceptable thoughts."

Her mother told Jill that people wouldn't like her if she were fat; she developed a history of anorexia and bulimia. She became very involved in athletics in junior high school. Already a mere size four or five dress size, Jill began to binge and starve. Laxative binges were routine from age nineteen to twenty-two. She suffered from painful menstrual cramps. She had nightmares about being responsible for too much and disappointing others. Jill craved bread. During her pregnancy, she often peeled lemons and ate them whole. She still loved sour lemonade, grapefruit, and pickles. She got diarrhea from whole milk or ice cream. What made Jill most memorable was her perpetual need to keep busy, busy, busy, quite a bit different from the all-or-nothing approach of Carl. The two share the characteristic of restlessness and high sexual energy, but their life experience is very different. Jill had to be touching, kissing, talking. She was compelled to be doing something every minute of her life.

We chose *Veratrum album* (White hellebore) for Jill because of her internal restlessness, impulse to touch and kiss others, hurriedness, tendency to menstrual cramps, diarrhea from dairy products, and her strong craving for sour foods. We saw her again three months later. She reported feeling much better beginning one week after she took the medicine. She told us, "My stomach hasn't

Veratrum album (white hellebore)

Individuals who need this medicine are usually intelligent, even precocious, and restless to the point of being ceaselessly busy. Children may engage in repetitive behaviors like stacking blocks or cutting and tearing things. *Veratrum* children are so restless that they never seem to stop, even to eat. They seem to know it all and can be bossy, self-righteous, and debative. Touching, hugging, and kissing inappropriately is common. Often chilly, they may have very cold hands and feet, which turn white or blue. Vomiting, diarrhea, and fainting are typical physical symptoms. They like cold food and drinks, ice, pickles, and fruit.

felt this good since I was twenty years old. I didn't even remember how good it could feel. I am so much more relaxed. The restlessness and hurriedness are much better and so is my hypersensitivity to the environment." Since receiving the two doses of *Veratrum,* Jill has felt much calmer despite the many stresses of her busy life.

The Dream Warrior

Rob was a 47-year-old chiropractor from California. He had been an oral surgeon and had also studied acupuncture, Oriental bodywork, reflexology, iridology, and Eastern philosophy. He was a black belt in martial arts and taught yoga classes. He had even prepared for a year to become a priest. Despite his busy practice, Rob meditated two hours a day. He described himself as "very goal-oriented and determined. My energy is normally very high, but I need a stimulus to get me going. I use herbal stimulants. I'm always having to know more, be more. I'm looking for total wholeness. I try to make people happy. I could easily give up my life for a cause or to save someone's life."

Rob was the life of the party and loved to do stand-up comedy acts. He enjoyed being center stage. "I've read a lot about amazing people like Michelangelo, Buddha, and great comedians, and I have wondered what makes them tick. Great comedians have cynical minds. So do I. I have a cutting humor, but I'm not malicious. The other day I was in an elevator with an overweight woman. The back of her jeans said, 'Guess'. I said to myself, '500 pounds'. I make flippant, ridiculous jokes about people as I go through my day, then I make friends with them later. I make friends very easily."

Rob thrived on helping people. "I can see 80 to 90 patients a day, then feel more energized. It's a sympathetic adrenaline high. I have a tendency to overdo things. I'm good at everything I do. I never stop to pat myself on back. My father always expected me to get 100 on every test. He'd criticize me if I got a 92 or a 95 and say nothing if I got 100. I was one of the top three ping-pong players in college. I'll do really well at something then I'll leave it." Rob had a history of using lots of recreational drugs, especially during his long period of travel in South America.

What Rob wanted most was help with his irritability. It was the one underlying problem that he had not been able to shake. In high school, he had gotten into many fights. "There were always fights. I didn't want to get into them because of all the blood and teeth. But I knew I somehow had to protect myself and others.Whenever I get into an argument with someone, I tend to hang on to it. I'd really like to be able to let go of my anger." Rob's grandfather told him that he had noticed Rob always wanted to defend his point. Rob was embarassed by his own anger. His father had a problem with anger, too.

There was something else very striking about Rob: his dreams. "My dreams have a continuous theme. I'm always fighting with someone, and I'm always the good guy, defending and helping people. I use hand-to-hand combat. Last week I had five dreams about fighting. I have them practically every night, sometimes several in one night. Most of the time I have to go correct something that's wrong. I wish these dreams would stop."

Rob also suffered from hemorrhoids and constipation. His joints popped too easily. He was very exercise-oriented and loved to run and work out. "I lose myself in it." He disliked being cold. Rob loved sweets and bread.

He "would go wild with dairy," even though he should have avoided it because dairy caused him to suffer from sinus congestion.

Although Rob had not been diagnosed with ADD, we recognized the impulsivity, daring quality, and his lack of follow through as typical characteristics of adults with ADD. He would pick up an area of study or work, plunge into it wholeheartedly, then drop it and go on to something else. He was one of the most intense and fascinating people we had ever met. Rob had a superhuman aspect. What would normally take several people entire lifetimes to achieve, Rob accomplished in half his lifetime. Activities that would exhaust the average person gave him more energy. He exhibited a ceaseless yearning for the experiences of life and a tireless desire to help others. Rob demonstrated a type of hyperfocus that we often see in people with ADD. Just as children become engrossed in Nintendo for hours on end, adults with ADD can focus intensely on one thing, but move quickly from one task, or career, to another due to their need for constant stimulation and change. They need to have high levels of challenge in their waking hours, and sometimes even during their dreams.

We gave Rob one dose of *Agaricus muscaria,* a type of mushroom used as a hallucinogen by indigenous groups in various parts of the world. It is a medicine for people that undertake tremendous exploits and who also experience episodes of rage during which they are capable of great feats of strength. It is not surprising that Rob had actually used this mushroom many times while traveling in South America.

At his six week follow-up visit, Rob told us, "I've never felt better. Before, I had dreams about conflict. I was always fighting with adversaries. I've only had these dreams a few times since taking the medicine. I haven't been irritable as much. My digestion is better."

Rob wrote us a letter five months later. "The medicine seems like the perfect match. I've had only two or three dreams of combat over the past five months. I used to have multiple combat dreams every single night. Gone! I hardly get angry anymore. I have more energy and I'm happier. I have more mental clarity, more focus, more purpose, and I feel closer to God. I'm also much less chilly. This is what you'd call a success story."

When we spoke with Rob by phone five months later, he reported, "I have lots of energy all the time. My dreams were fatiguing me. I always had to protect people. I'm talking about three, four, five battles a night. Sometimes I'd wake in the middle because my life was in danger, then I'd go back to sleep and renew the dream. I've had only three battle dreams since you gave me the medicine a year ago. Everything in my life has improved. I'm much more balanced and not as intense all the time. I'm more laid back, yet much more focused in general. My irritability has diminished tremendously. My hemorrhoids have only flared up a couple of times over the past year. I no longer have gas or bloating. Zero. My joints pop a lot less. I'm blossoming."

Rob has not needed another dose of the *Agaricus* since the original dose.

"I'm Scattered. It's Hard to Get on Track"

Genevieve, age forty, had never been formally diagnosed with ADD, but many of her symptoms match the diagnostic criteria. She came to us primarily for her digestive problems, but also complained repeatedly about poor the reasons why I'm so stressed, but I just can't handle them. There are so many demands, so many things for me to juggle. My husband and I misunderstand each other. We don't communicate well so there's friction.

"I'm scattered and have a hard time focusing. I have a good heart and my intentions are right, but there's so much going on. I'm constantly jumping from one thing to another. It's not new. It's the modus operandi that I've used for a long time. I like change, variety, people. But I'd like to be more centered instead of a feather in the wind or a butterfly. Before I had children, I used to just move whenever I felt like it. I must have lived in seventeen different places in Arizona in just a couple of years. Then I went back and forth to Central America.

"I really need harmony. I need to be in a better state of balance, but I don't want to be a patient of anyone for long. My track record of sticking with things isn't very good. My husband's always telling me to finish what I start. I get too fragmented. I constantly feel like I'm failing in every area of my life. I feel fragmented when I even talk about my life. I'm not very good at organizing things. I've bought so many organizers that I could open a second-hand store."

Genevieve had been diagnosed with diverticulosis (the formation of pouches in the lining of the small intestine), which caused her to feel bloated much of the time. She came for help with her digestive problems and had no idea that homeopathy could help her mind as well.

What we perceived as Genevieve's greatest limitation was her mental fragmentation and her inability to complete anything. She was indeed just like a feather blowing in the wind, previously from home to home and continent to continent, most recently from one thought or idea to the next. We felt that the characteristics unique to Genevieve were: undertaking many things, yet persevering in nothing; inconstancy; and persisting in nothing. We gave Genevieve *Plantago* (Plantain).

People needing plant medicines are often plant-like. Plants are sensitive, gentle, diffuse, changeable, and move with the wind. This was definitely Genevieve's nature. Those needing *Plantago* can also be very confused, so restless and nervous that they pace back and forth, and do work hastily. The description "hurry or haste in occupation; desire to do several things at once, but cannot finish anything" appears in the homeopathic literature under *Plantago* and certainly seems to depict Genevieve perfectly.

Genevieve returned five weeks later to say that she felt much better. "The first thing that I noticed was that I felt calmer, more patient. I was able to take a deep breath and be more still. I think I've found a centered place.

"I remember to write things down now. I'm clearer. I pick up more on details and am able to accomplish more. I'm not feeling as chaotic. I'm staying on track despite the fact that a lot of things have been going on. Although it's the nature of a mother to jump from one thing to another, I'm handling it better. I don't get frustrated as easily. My outbursts are really rare now. I used to get really upset over things I couldn't make go the way I wanted. My inner voice is talking louder and more clearly now."

The only time we had prescribed *Plantago* before was for dental pain, for which it had worked quite well. When Genevieve came for this first return visit, she mentioned that her teeth had been hurting quite a bit until she took the medicine. Now the pain was gone.

17

"I Have to Tell Him Everything Ten Times"

Distractibility and Difficulty Concentrating

He Cannot Hang On to Directions

Grace brought in her son Jeff when he was eight. He was under evaluation for ADD at the local children's hospital because of his inability to sit still and pay attention in the classroom. Kindergarten had been a nightmare for Jeff. His attitude was terrible; staying in his seat was impossible. Jeff jumped up every few minutes to sharpen pencils or chatter with his friends. Anything and everything distracted him. His mind drifted constantly. His mother told us, "He can even hear the grass grow." Jeff simply could not hang on to directions. He talked out in class on a regular basis. His teachers lost patience with Jeff because of his interruptions and inability to focus. Jeff was quite a storyteller. He would also conveniently forget to tell his mother when he got into trouble at school. His academic abilities were a real problem. He was held back in the first grade because he could not read. When we first saw Jeff, he had just started the second grade and was writing his numbers and letters backwards.

Jeff's parents divorced when he was three. It was an awful time for him. He continued to act like a baby for several years. Jeff did not want to stop nursing. He was very insecure, "a momma's boy." He became frightened very easily. He acted in a charming, sweet manner with adults and younger children, but he was shy with kids his age. Jeff had a very hard time making friends. He was afraid to try anything new. He could never get enough attention and always insisted, "Watch me, watch me!"

Jeff experienced enormous mood swings. His mother described his as "happy as a lark or mad as a hornet." He cried, screamed, swore, slammed doors, and alternately told his mother that he loved and hated her. When he was angry, he became wild, throwing things on the floor and ripping up paper.

Life was scary for Jeff. He was afraid to look out of the windows at night. He slept in bed with his brother until recently because he was afraid to be alone. Jeff held his mother's hand while watching scary movies until he was seven. He did not like the dark and slept with a night light.

He complained of diarrhea, stomach aches, and a constant runny nose. He loved chicken, sweets, and hamburgers. Jeff became wound up and wild after eating sugar. His ears and face turned bright red and he could not stop talking.

The medicine that benefited Jeff the most was *Lycopodium* (Club moss). This medicine can help fearful children who act immaturely and try to cover up their mistakes. They make every effort to appear courageous and powerful, but inside they are timid and afraid. Kids like Jeff often feel more comfortable playing with younger children rather than their peers, because they feel older and can boss the younger children around. These children are very concerned with what others think and try to look cool at all costs. A deep insecurity inside often causes them to feel very anxious about performing in public or taking examinations where their inner weakness or lack of mastery might be revealed. There may also be a tendency to dyslexia and distractibility. These children often go wild for sweets but can also have a bad reaction to sugar, physically or behaviorally.

Two months after he was given the medicine, Jeff got his highest marks ever in school. His dyslexia was improving. He was able to sit still, raise his hand, and pay attention in class. Over the next eighteen months, Jeff's behavior steadily improved. He was able to make new friends more

Lycopodium clavatum (club moss)

Those needing this medicine are often fearful and cowardly but try not to show it. Inside they feel inadequate and lack self-confidence, often having been raised by parents who constantly put them down and tell them they cannot do anything right. These children boss others around, especially children younger than themselves, and may even assume the role of the class clown. These children can be distractible and dyslexic. People needing *Lycopodium* are reluctant to try new things because they fear they will fail. The most prominent food craving is sweets and there is a tendency toward hypoglycemia. Physical symptoms often include gas and bloating, particularly from beans and the cabbage family.

easily. The other children started to look up to Jeff because he was so agile in physical education. He acted less impulsively and his teachers reported that he was extremely well behaved. He accomplished two years of math in six months. For the first time, the teachers recognized that Jeff was very bright. They removed him from special education classes where had been placed due to his unruly behavior. Now, three years after beginning homeopathy, he continues to do very well in a regular classroom.

A Sweet Kid Who Just Could Not Pay Attention

Michael was diagnosed with ADD at age six. His pediatrician prescribed Ritalin, but his mother was not comfortable with medicating her child. She brought in a copy of Michael's scores on the Conners' Rating Scales. Michael was shown to have very significant difficulties with squirminess, pouting, and sulking, worrying about others, making inappropriate noises, disturbing other children, restlessness in the classroom, and immature behavior. Next on his list of unacceptable behaviors were excitability and impulsivity, sucking or chewing, frequent crying, distractibility, frustrated easily, boasting and bragging, demanding nature, hypersensitivity to criticism, daydreaming, excessive demands for teacher's attention, submissiveness, and failure to complete tasks.

Test scores made it appear that Michael had significant learning and behavior problems, but the child we saw in our office was sweet and sensitive. His mother described him as "pretty darn average. He's like any other six-year-old kid, but more active." He definitely had difficulty sitting still in school. His work was

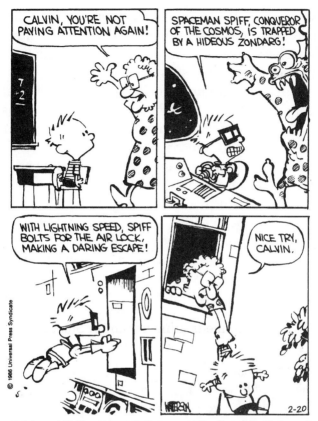

Calvin and Hobbes © (1986) Watterson. Distributed by Universal Press Syndicate. Reprinted with permission. All rights reserved.

inconsistent. "Some of his papers were done perfectly, others looked like an alien did them." He preferred to socialize rather than do his homework. The feedback from teachers was that his behavior was fantastic one day and really bad the next.

Michael became wound up very easily, especially when he felt bored. He would crumple up little scraps of paper and throw them away one at a time. He needed to be in constant movement. He sometimes ran out of the classroom eight to ten times a day to go to the bathroom. Michael often crawled around on the floor in class. To make matters worse, he would not stop after the teacher reprimanded him the first time.

His mother found it difficult to get Michael to focus at home. If the television were on or the curtains open, she had to make him repeat back what she told him or he would not respond. Michael was never violent or aggressive and tended to be a follower. Kids loved him because they thought he was funny, but his self-confidence was really low.

Michael's parents divorced when he was two years old. He was never sure when his dad would come pick him up. He was a pleaser. He worried about his father's violence toward his stepmother, about being late for school, about his shoelaces breaking, and about having enough money for lunch. He was preoccupied with who would pick him up from school and how many days he would stay with his dad.

A very sensitive child, Michael cried if reprimanded even gently. "It scares me when somebody yells at me. I'm afraid I'll have to be on restriction again. I get really

Natrum muriaticum (sodium chloride)

The main feeling in *Natrum muriaticum,* derived from table salt, is being rejected and unloved, and withdrawing in order to protect oneself. These children are usually shy, bookish, and introverted. They cry their salty tears alone, not wanting to be embarrassed in public. They often become confidantes to one of their parents or to friends. Headaches, allergies, and cold sores are common complaints. They often crave salt, pasta, and bread, and are averse to slimy foods and fat.

upset at myself." Michael really wanted to be good and felt very bad about himself when he messed up and got into trouble.

We found many seeming contradictions in Michael. He was disruptive and inappropriate, yet highly sensitive. He could be very sulky or very loving. He was very scared about making mistakes, yet went ahead and acted out anyway. Many of his symptoms were classic ADD symptoms which did not differentiate him from the many other children diagnosed with ADD, such as impulsivity, excitability, distractibility, and difficulty maintaining his focus. Yet, unlike many children with ADD, he felt very guilty about his unacceptable behaviors and constantly worried about "messing up." Most children who are naughty are not overly sensitive pleasers as Michael was. It was this combination of typical ADD symptoms and oversensitive and excessive worrying that stood out about Michael in our eyes.

Michael responded extremely well to one dose of *Natrum muriaticum.* This medicine is given to very sensitive people, often after an experience of grief or loss. People needing this medicine are unusually sensitive to reprimands, and tend to feel very bad about themselves when they have done something wrong. Michael has needed this medicine only two times over the past year. Within several weeks of beginning treatment, Michael's teachers were amazed at the tremendous improvement in his attitude and behavior. His continual movement had diminished. Before homeopathic treatment, Michael received four to five checks (corresponding to reprimands) a day. By his follow-up visit six weeks after starting homeopathy, he had not received even one check. Michael was no longer so sensitive to reprimands.

When we asked Michael how he felt, he replied, "It's easier to concentrate. Sometimes I'm getting stars and superstars and Mommy's really proud of me." What was most touching about seeing the changes in Michael was how much better he felt about himself.

Michael's improvement has continued. He no longer acts out in class or at lunch. He stays in his seat more and does not worry as much. His leadership skills have improved tremendously. He was recently chosen "student of the week." The biggest improvement the teacher has noticed is his effort. Everyone is just thrilled with Michael's behavior.

He Gets Sidetracked from a Simple Command

Shawn's preschool teacher recommended that his hearing be tested at age three because of his difficulty listening. When his hearing proved normal, he was put on Dexedrine. The medication speeded him up, caused him to be "emotionally distraught," and resulted in bedwetting.

When Shawn was six, his mother decided to try homeopathy. It was hard for him to sit still in class. His attention span was short. He got sidetracked very easily from even a simple command. He was unable to focus on the teacher's instructions. Shawn was extremely impatient. If not allowed to do something, he became very upset and would not listen to reason. He talked loudly and became carried away easily. He loved television and hated going to bed.

Shawn's behavior was erratic. He was affectionate one minute and aggressive the next. He was not good at following rules when he played games with other children. He had trouble mingling with them and had a tendency to push them. When they did something to him, he retaliated by hitting and kicking. When he became really angry, he screamed, threatened to hit everyone, and told them he hated them.

Shawn always had one habit or another. He bit his nails to the extreme when younger. Later he grabbed at his genitals. Now he picked his nose habitually. He also stuttered.

He was a very creative child. He loved Halloween because of the skeletons, witches, ghosts, bats, and scarecrows, even though he was afraid of them.

What was most outstanding about Shawn was his excessive, erratic nature. Everything Shawn did was extreme, whether talking, staying up too late, lashing out at others, or picking his nose.

We treated Shawn with *Medorrhinum,* the same medicine described earlier in the case of Carl, one of the adults with ADD. Two months later, Shawn's mother reported that he had much less anger and was no longer hitting his brother. His concentration was much improved. He could now focus on tasks and could sit through church without wiggling. He was not nearly as impatient and could entertain himself while waiting for an hour. He was reading and sleeping better. One year after he started homeopathic treatment, Shawn's mother reported that he was a normal kid. Since the homeopathy, he had done very well in school and has gotten along fine with the other children. He has not needed another dose of the *Medorrhinum.*

18

"She Can't Sit Still for Even a Minute"
Excessive Restlessness and Impulsivity

A Teenager on the Go Go Go

Sixteen-year-old Sherrie was referred to us by her family practice physician because of a five-year history of ADD. She had been on Ritalin since the sixth grade. In kindergarten Sherrie was sent out of the classroom for talking too much. An aunt and a cousin on both sides of the family had also been diagnosed as hyperactive. Her father and maternal aunt suffered from manic depression. Without her Ritalin, she was unable to focus. Easily distracted by noise or movement, Sherrie found it very difficult to concentrate while taking tests. Paying attention in conversation was also a challenge. Sherrie complained of talking without listening and often found herself staring off into space in mid-sentence. No matter how much she told herself to be quiet, she blurted out her thoughts or feelings anyway. It was embarrassing at times, though much of the time she had little, if any, awareness of how she affected other people. Sherrie was used to her friends asking her to be quiet. She had a reputation among her friends of acting immaturely and of being the last one to catch on to a joke. While driving, she often daydreamed. She would become confused when she saw a car in another lane, as if she did not believe she was seeing it.

Sherrie was very antsy, always fidgeting and fiddling. Clicking her nails against her teeth and tapping her fingers was a perpetual occupation. Sherrie's poking, hugging, and pulling at other people was a constant annoyance to them, but she could not keep her hands to herself. Sherrie was always moving some part of her body. She would skip down the hall to release her pent-up energy. Without having a way to let it out, she felt that she would scream. "The energy is trapped inside of me and has to be pushed out. It's all out of control," she explained.

Ritalin gave Sherrie hives and made her feel like she did not know herself. Her habit of being "a major procrastinator" was not affected by the Ritalin. With or without medication, she asked lots of "dumb questions" even though she maintained a 3.8 grade-point average.

Sherrie had a passion for pickles. She ate them straight from the jar. She also liked to suck on ice. Her fingers and toes became extremely cold when she skied.

Sherrie's defining features were her extreme restlessness and ceaseless activity. We gave her *Veratrum album,* mentioned earlier in Jill's case of adult ADD. Again notice the strong desire for sour foods. These people are generally good-natured and helpful but overexuberant. Their energy oozes out around the edges. As is frequently the case in treating children, we gave Sherrie a single dose of the medicine and asked her to return in five weeks.

When we saw her again, she was very happy with her progress. She had informed her psychiatrist that she wanted to discontinue the Ritalin before taking the homeopathic medicine. When she came for her follow-up visit, Sherrie found our parking lot without directions, something she could normally do only with the help of Ritalin. Her grades were better, in contrast to her previous efforts to discontinue Ritalin, when her grades plummeted to all F's.

Her parents also reported that Sherrie's behavior had drastically improved. She no longer stared blankly. Her friends told her that she "wasn't as crazy" as she used to be. No longer antsy, she felt a lot more controlled. The urge to poke, hug, and pull at other people had stopped plaguing her. Sherrie's leg no longer moved restlessly, nor was she clicking her nails against her teeth. Sherrie remarked that she was not as depressed as she had been, although she had not actually described herself that way previously.

Sherrie now had "a real appetite" instead of sporadic urges. She no longer experienced "that special taste for pickles." Sherrie needed two doses of the *Veratrum* over the next year and a half, then discontinued treatment because she felt well. She did not resume taking Ritalin. As her treatment progressed, Sherrie was able to notice whenever she felt even a little hyperactive and could stop it by telling herself to relax. Before beginning homeopathic treatment, Sherrie had been unable to notice or control her behavior patterns. Now she became fidgety only once in a while instead of all the time. When her voice became loud, she quieted down, which was also impossible in the past. "It's like somebody opened the curtains and let me see."

The Didgeridoo Kid from Down Under

Angela's mother brought her to see us when she was twenty-two months old. The Australian family was visiting the United States during Angela's father's didgeridoo concert tour. The didgeridoo is a rhythmic Aboriginal instrument. Angela had a red rash on her face. She had not gotten one good night's sleep (nor had her parents!) since birth. When her mother weaned her at seven months, Angela refused cow's milk. Angela had a pattern of waking in the middle of the night crying, distressed, and disoriented. Her parents tried to soothe her despair by letting her sleep with them; otherwise she woke repeatedly crying for her mother. She fought for hours against going to sleep. Her mother described her as being "in a frenzy every night." Angela's exhausted parents had even resorted unsuccessfully to giving their little darling sleeping pills.

Angela was extremely willful. It was extremely nerve wracking to travel with her, which was a conflict with her father's entertainment career. Angela screamed at the top of her lungs during most of our interview with her. She became inconsolable. Even when her mother offered her a bottle of her favorite juice, she refused. She had the habit of throwing herself on the floor when unhappy.

Angela loved people. She was a very lively baby and did not want to nap. She lived in a busy household where friends and family members were always coming and going. She had walked at nine months and ran at ten. She climbed fearlessly on anything within her reach. She loved playing with animals and putting on her mother's lipstick. When we inquired about Angela's musical affinity, her mother told us that as soon as the music came on, Angela squirmed and danced. Even at her very young age, she sat at the piano bench and tried to bang on the keys. She loved to play her father's guitar when he held her on his knee. Family friends often commented on the child's rhythmical talents.

Angela had been diagnosed with an unusual skin condition called dermatomyositis, which showed up as purplish, red, scarred areas on her fingers resembling tiny splinters.

We gave Angela one dose of homeopathic *Tarentula.* This medicine, made from the Spanish spider, is for over-active children who are extremely lively, love to be the center of attention, climb like little spiders, and love dancing and rhythmic music. They can have tantrums and fits and often have a mischievous, manipulative quality. It is understandable that Angela, raised in an environment of music and dance, needed this lively medicine. A well-respected Italian homeopathic physician, Massimo Mangialavori, recounts a story of a small southern village in

Tarentula hispanica (tarantula spider)

Tarentula children have rhythm. Their active, climbing, jumping restlessness mimics animal behavior. They love music and rhythmic activities like dancing, tapping, or drumming, and it soothes them. Cunning and mischievous, they play tricks on their parents and other children, tell lies, and love to hide. They are very hurried and impatient. Often destructive, they have to be watched very closely, as they are capable of breaking anything they get their hands on. They are very impulsive and distractible. Twitching and jerking of the muscles is a common symptom. They are often attracted to bright colors.

Italy near the seaport of Tarent. A group of girls in the village suffered from a hysterical type of insanity which was only relieved when they danced in a type of frenzy and cut with knives or swords.[3] Although it did not come up in Angela's case, many children needing *Tarentula* do have an urge to wildly cut clothing and other things during their rages.

Angela's mother called from Australia five weeks after she took the medicine. Angela had no further tantrums or extreme moodiness; "just the odd two-year-old stuff." Her mother had no complaints about Angela's behavior compared to before she took the *Tarentula*. Now she was much more easily managed when she became upset. She jumped up and down occasionally when her mother said no, but would settle down. Angela was much more easily entertained. It was much easier for her to sit in a car, which had been a major problem previously. Her teeth grinding, which her mother forgot to mention in the first interview, was 90 percent improved. The redness and scarring on her hands were also better. Angela's mother added that prior to the homeopathy, her daughter was forever tapping, teasing, and getting into mischief. These behaviors had also improved. "Looks like Miss Spider's working," her mother exclaimed.

Angela needed one more dose of the *Tarentula* five months later because some of her symptoms had returned, though to a much lesser degree than before the homeopathic treatment. Angela's dermatologist was quite surprised that the redness and inflammation of her fingers had improved significantly.

---

[3] Pelt, M., "Spiders in Nature and Homeopathy: Mangialavore in Wageningen, Autumn 1993 and 1994," *Homeopathic Links*, 8(3), 1995, p. 45-46.

The Little Girl Who Couldn't Sit Still

Six-year-old Sumi was a very cute little girl with honey-colored hair, green eyes, and gold skin. Her striking features resulted from her Japanese and Northern European heritage. We first interviewed Sumi and her family at a poolside table at a California hotel where we were speaking at a conference on homeopathy. What was most notable about Sumi was that she could not sit still for more than five minutes. She ran around the table, became easily distracted by the children in the swimming pool, or whispered something into her mother's ear. It seemed literally impossible for her to stay in one place.

Sumi was calm and sweet when she was an infant. She had suffered from ear infections, debilitating diarrhea, profuse perspiration, and lethargy. Sumi's speech was delayed. Her mother sought out homeopathic treatment for her now because of her restlessness. Sumi kissed, poked, prodded, and pulled. She was very affectionate. She blurted things out loudly. School was a struggle because of her difficulty concentrating, following directions, and staying at her desk. She wandered around and was always busy. Her verbal skills lagged far behind the other children at her grade level. It was particularly hard for her to remember words.

This sweet child seemed to lack any awareness of how her behavior affected others. She often came on too strongly, but did not realize it. She bit her nails down to the quick and even nibbled her toenails. Sumi loved cucumbers and liked to chew on ice.

Sumi may sound very similar to Sherrie and Jill, because of her relentless motion. They all needed the same medicine, *Veratrum album*. We first treated Sumi two and a half years ago. She is literally a different child now. Just weeks after starting homeopathy, Sumi began making excellent progress with her speech. She spent less time searching for words and her focus was greatly improved. She did not stumble or rush so much. Before she could only color one page at a time in a coloring book; within three weeks of taking the *Veratrum,* she was completing eight pages.

Over time, Sumi's progress continued. Her nailbiting diminished. She no longer kissed all the time. Her actions became more purposeful and centered and she became more aware of her impact on others. Sumi's teachers no longer complained about her disruptive behavior. Rather than the word-salad she used to communicate previously, now she could connect phrases and her vocabulary was growing. She remembered the names of her classmates whereas before she had been oblivious to such details. Sumi's parents were pleasantly surprised that she could handle kindergarten so well. During the next year, she grew five inches. Now, three years after starting homeopathy, Sumi is doing extremely well in all areas of her life.

One curious aspect of homeopathic treatment is what is called a return of old symptoms. This means that a particular symptom that an individual had in the past may briefly reappear in the process of healing. This occurred with Sumi. She briefly developed a small swelling in her breast just as she did at two months of age when she developed a breast bud. Her mother reported that it was at this time that her health problems originally began. During the course of homeopathic treatment, Sumi also broke out once in large blisters on her right ribs and back. They looked a lot like shingles. Sumi's mother had had herpes during her pregnancy. Both of these skin eruptions might seem like coincidence to the average person, but to the homeopath they are recognizable as a return of old symptoms, which is often necessary for deep and lasting healing.

19

"If I Say Black, He Says White"
Oppositional Behavior

All children have their stubborn moments. Some children
have their stubborn years. The children in this chapter are
more than strong-willed, let-me-do-it kids. They are
downright defiant. They do not respond to the most skill-
ful distraction techniques and generally drive their parents crazy by refusing to do almost anything that they are
asked. A sibling suggests one restaurant, an oppositional
child will insist on another. Even the simplest of tasks or
events like getting dressed for school or eating dinner can
become major battlegrounds. Children who are oppositional often wear their parents to a frazzle. They take the
lyric "I say potayto, you say potahto" to extremes.

According to conventional child psychology models, there are two categories of negative behaviors. The
first grouping is noncompliance, which includes not following directions, disregarding requests, or doing the
opposite of what is asked. This may include almost any
negative behavior such as tantrums, whining, breath
holding, and physical or verbal aggression.[4] The second

[4]Carolyn S. Schroeder and Betty N. Gordon, *Assessment and
Treatment of Childhood Problems* (New York: The Guilford Press,
1991), 273.

category, aggressive behavior, will be covered in the next chapter.

Oppositional Defiant Disorder, the official label for defiant children, is characterized by the frequent occurrence of the following behaviors: losing one's temper; arguing with adults; actively defying or refusing adult requests or rules; deliberately doing things that annoy other people; blaming others for his or her own mistakes; touchy or easily annoyed by others; angry and resentful; spiteful or vindictive; swears or uses obscene language.[5]

Each of the following children matches this categorization, but each youngster is unique. It is this uniqueness that allows the homeopath to select a specific medicine for each child.

"I Try to Be Good But My Head Doesn't Let Me"

Darin, age five, had been diagnosed with ADD one month before his parents called us. They had opted to try Ritalin first. The medication did improve his concentration, but his mother preferred a more natural alternative.

Darin smiled as the interview began. His mother explained that he had difficulty following instructions. Darin's mother home-schooled him, but she couldn't seem to find a teaching approach that worked for him. Both mother and son became frustrated on a regular basis. When she told us that he had started daycare at three, Darin corrected her. "No, I was two." He did not have a good time playing by himself. He needed a lot of reassurance that he was being good or doing the right

---

[5] Ibid., 279.

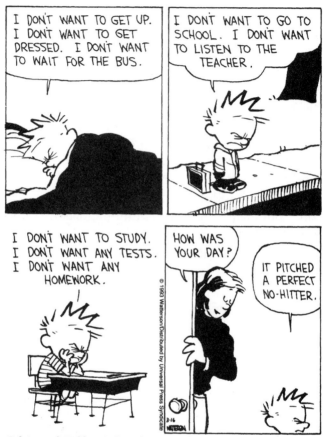

Calvin and Hobbes © (1993) Watterson. Distributed by Universal Press Syndicate. Reprinted with permission. All rights reserved.

thing. He frequently asked his mother, "Am I being good?" or "Am I being quiet?" Darin often told his mother, "I try to be good, to do the right thing, but my head doesn't let me."

Darin had problems listening and following rules. His mother had to ask him again and again to do things. He just didn't seem to act on her requests. Specific problem areas were being unable to settle down at night to go to sleep, to stay quiet, and to stop bothering his brother.

"Darin gets really unhappy when he's reprimanded. It makes him cry. He just wants to be good. It takes time for him to settle down at night. I have to go in three times and eventually spank him five nights out of seven to get him to go to sleep. The wrestling, kicking, and hitting are hard to stop.

"The feedback from school is that he has difficulty settling down for structured activities. He is unable to sit still, messes with his neighbors, and has a blatant disregard for direct requests." Darin argued constantly, even over the simplest issues. He always engaged in dialogue. His mother elaborated: "Yesterday he saw some cookies. I told him he needed to wait until lunch to eat them. He kept asking me about it for five minutes. He tells me when he thinks something is unfair. If I say 'white,' he says 'black,' even when we discuss the littlest things. He'll be certain that he's right. It's very tiring for me. He wants things his way and loses it if they're not. He breaks into tears at the drop of a hat."

Enthusiastic but impatient, Darin could not wait for things to happen. He demanded affection in an almost frantic, anxious way. His mother described it as a desperate feeling. He clung to her and did not want her to read or talk to anyone else. When he traveled, he fidgeted and pestered his brother. When he spent time with his dad, from whom his mother was divorced, he called his mother after only a few hours to complain that he missed her and wanted to go home.

Darin was anxious and insecure, fearful, but determined. He wanted to learn to ride his bicycle without training wheels from the very start. He was afraid of the dark and sleeping alone and had scary dreams.

When we asked Darin's mother about her pregnancy, she explained that she was very unhappy throughout the pregnancy. She felt frustrated and vulnerable about having to rely on Darin's father who was irresponsible. She missed the security of having family around and kept fantasizing about moving to Hawaii to be with her parents. We asked her whether Darin was more like her or his dad. She felt Darin was very similar to his father who didn't like to be by himself or to do things alone. He was always on the move and was a chronic procrastinator. Both father and son were reckless and accident-prone. Neither paid attention to where they were going.

Darin's only physical complaints were bumpy rashes on his hips and occasional headaches. His face was always pale, his ears red, and he had chronic puffiness under his eyes.

What was most unusual about Darin? His difficulty concentrating? His refusal to do what his mother asked? His unwillingness to settle down at night? Pestering his brother? All of these characteristics are very common in many children with ADD. What really stood out in our eyes was Darin's oppositional nature, his strong response to being reprimanded or talked about, and the theme of homesickness in both Darin and in his mother. The medicine that best matches that combination of symptoms is *Capsicum* (Red pepper). Again we gave Darin a single dose.

Darin's mother brought him back to see us two months later. "It was a gradual change. He's calmer. He's talking more and able to work things out better. My son's appetite is good and he's more willing to try new things. He's no longer asking if he's being good or quiet and there aren't as many arguments. He's more reasonable and rarely says the opposite. If I tell him he can't do something, he won't argue. He still pouts, but he gets over it easily. Maybe he's a little on the defiant side, but he becomes reasonable very quickly. There's been a gradual easing into being more agreeable. He's still impatient and sensitive to scolding and sad situations, but he's much more appropriate about demanding attention. Darin's also less clingy and possessive. He was unhappy for a few days about my starting to work, but now he's fine with it."

Darin had no more scary dreams. He had not talked about wanting to go home while visiting his father. His headaches were gone as well as the bumpy rashes on his hips. He continued to do quite well for over a year and did not need a repetition of the *Capsicum*. At that time the family moved to another state and requested that we send his records to a homeopathic clinic nearby.

"You're a Mean, Bad Mommy!"

Five-year-old Ben had sandy-brown hair, freckles, and a mischievous grin. His parents were at their wits' end when they brought him to us because of his extreme disobedience. Ben would not listen to his parents despite their efforts at numerous parenting techniques. Whenever his mother or father asked him to do something, he balked. There was absolutely no reasoning with him. If his parents told him, "You can't," he became hysterical, screamed, cried, and threw whatever was in his vicinity. He engaged in slugging matches with his mother in public which embarrassed her terribly. He yelled, "I'm not afraid of you. It's not fair. You're a mean, bad mommy." Ben's defiance knew no limits.

Ben did not get along well with other children. He pushed and hit them, but when they did it back to him he told them it was not fair. He liked to wrestle and play karate and insisted on taking charge whenever he played with other children. Ben was terrible with animals. His parents had to tell him ten times a day to stop tormenting the cat and dog. It took Ben thirty to forty-five minutes to get dressed in the morning. He stopped and started over and over again and asked questions incessantly, driving his parents crazy.

Ben was a precocious child. He was bold and relished climbing on high surfaces. He chattered for hours on end. Loud noises really bothered him. He was fixated on violence, weapons, and alien movies. Ben's moods could go from black to white in a matter of seconds, as if something snapped inside of him. When angry, he told his parents that he didn't want them to look at him or touch him. If others were injured, sometimes he was sympathetic and at other times he laughed. Ben talked very loudly and was extremely obstinate.

Ben complained of painful warts on his left foot and of growing pains. He was a restless sleeper and flailed his arms and legs in bed. He often woke upside down. He picked his nose and ground his teeth frequently. Ben loved noodles and sweets. He had an enormous appetite and often complained that he was "hungry to death."

Cina (wormseed)

Cross is the middle name of children needing *Cina*. They can be among the most irritable of children for no good reason. They do not seem to know what they want and reject what they are given. They want to be rocked but they do not like to be carried (except over the shoulder), touched, or looked at. They pinch, kick, and hit out of irritability and contradiction. Worms are a causative factor in some cases, especially pinworms. Children pick or bore into their nose or ears, scratch their bottoms, and grind their teeth at night. Serious cases may include convulsions.

We gave Ben a homeopathic medicine that is very useful for cross, irritable, contrary children who pick their noses and bottoms and grind their teeth. They are fussy, obstinate, throw tantrums, and do not want to be touched when mad. The medicine is derived from a plant named *Cina* (Wormseed). These children sometimes have a history of pinworms or other parasites.

Ben had a dramatic response to homeopathy. When his mother called six weeks after we gave him a dose of *Cina,* she was delighted to report that the warts on the soles of his foot were completely gone. His teeth-grinding had decreased considerably. Most importantly, Ben's behavior was much better. "Now he's your normal, average kid." There had been no more slugging matches with his mom and no more temper tantrums. Ben was less defiant. To his mother's relief, he no longer told her that she was mean and bad. His nose-picking was much better. He was not as fixated on violence. His bones did not ache anymore. He did not complain about being touched. Ben needed one more dose of the *Cina* ten weeks later, then continued to do well. His noise sensitivity diminished considerably so that even a chain saw did not bother him.

Ben's mother gave birth to a second child five years later. She called us for help because of the baby's voracious appetite, shrieking, and fussiness. His little brother needed *Chamomilla,* a medicine quite similar to *Cina.*

"No! No! No!"

Davey was a seven-year-old, lanky, delicate, fair-skinned child. He was significantly delayed developmentally and had been late to roll, crawl, and lift his head. Walking was delayed until age two and his vocabulary was still very limited. The child's stamina was low as was his self-confidence.

His mom was very challenged by his behavior. He darted from one thing to another and loved to run outside, even down the street by himself when his mother had her back turned. He got a rise out of teasing others and even hit them to see how they would react. Davey was quick to kick others if they bugged him. He had a mind of his own and was hard to discipline. He did not listen well. An impulsive child, he had trouble keeping his hands off of things. When Davey threw a tantrum, he often struck out at whomever was standing closest.

Frequently quite obstinate and naughty, Davey repeatedly tested the limits that his mother tried to set for him. He threw a yelling, screaming fit whenever she tried to put him to bed or bathe him. He often hit his head or bit his hand out of frustration. Impatience came to him easily and he would insist, "Mama, go, go, go." He was always in a rush, and would grab his mother's arm to make her move faster. When in the car, he would insist that his mother move on when she stopped at a red light. Davey's mother lamented, "He won't listen to anything I say. He does what he pleases. He yells 'no' or screeches, defies directions, and whines a lot. When he gets upset he doesn't want me to touch him."

Davey bit his nails and picked his nose. He had a persistent rash and chronic, deep coughs. He could never get his fill of ice cream and raw cookie dough.

Davey presented a number of problems, but what most bothered his mother was his defiance and obstinacy. The medicine that most helped Davey was homeopathic *Tuberculinum,* a useful medicine for thin children who throw tantrums and have chronic coughs. They love to go outside and to travel and often hit, kick, and bite others. They often have the characteristic of destroying their parents' prized possessions. Davey's behavior improved considerably during the year we gave him *Tuberculinum*. He was not as frustrated and combative. He did not hit as he had previously. His mother described him as "a delight to be around." He became more cuddly. He was still bossy but not defiant. He got into trouble much less. His hitting, kicking, and biting improved, as did the rash. Davey is an example of a child who will always face significant challenges due to his developmental disability, but his attitude and behavior changed substantially for the better with homeopathy each time he received the medicine.

Tuberculinum (nosode)

Never satisfied and desiring constant change, children needing *Tuberculinum* like to travel. Often allergic to cats and other animal dander, they also can have a strong fear of cats and animals and be mean to them. They are irritable and mean to other children, and can break their parents' favorite things just to get back at them or can be generally destructive, even of their own toys. These children can be very restless. They can also be sensitive, artistic, and very bright. *Tuberculinum* children are prone to respiratory complaints such as allergies, asthma, and pneumonia. They look thin and pale, with swollen glands. Children sometimes have dark hair on their spine and can be prone to scoliosis and birth defects. They desire cold milk, fat, ice cream, pork, and smoked meat.

20

---cᗺᗡᗷᗺᗞ---

"I'm Gonna Chop His Head Off"
Violence and Rage

Adults and children alike are shocked and often terrified at the recent epidemic of violence in the United States. Violent crimes perpetrated by and against children, previously unthinkable in this country, are now commonplace. In certain neighborhoods of Los Angeles and other cities where gang activity is rampant, children may be in danger of losing their lives on the school playgrounds or in their own backyards.

A number of cases of matricide and patricide have been reported over the past few years, these incidents are often a result of physical or sexual abuse by the parents toward the children. Laws have been changed so that minors who are convicted of murder receive the same punishment as adults.

Two shocking front page articles in *Seattle Times* were entitled: "Fed-up teachers head to court" and "Grim herald in L.A. school yard: the 'shooting bell.'"[6] The first article reported a yearlong incident in a Kentucky Spanish class in which one disruptive child

---

[6]*Seattle Times*, September 18, 1995.

instructed his classmates to speak every day in class about different methods of murder. When school officials reprimanded the child with only a forty-minute detention period, the teacher went to juvenile court, got a restraining order, and filed a complaint of terroristic threatening. The teacher then sued the child. He was ordered to pay $8,700 for her emotional stress and medical bills as well as $25,000 in punitive damages. After winning her suit, the Spanish teacher, who had taught for twenty-five years, retired to avoid future confrontations. She vowed to use the money she won to set up a trust fund for teachers who are threatened or harassed. Spokespeople for the American Federation of Teachers and the Seattle and Washington Education associations say this is by no means the only such case and that teachers are demanding control of their classrooms rather than being intimidated by fear.

The second article told of a special bell at a Langdon Avenue elementary school in Los Angeles that alerted children to violence just outside the school building and sent them ducking for cover. The students were trained to return to class when the "shooting bell" stopped ringing. The school was located in the North Hills neighborhood where there were constant shoot-outs between members of vying Hispanic gangs.

In the same newspaper appeared still another story about a three-year-old girl who was slain when her parents' car took a wrong turn in Los Angeles. Gang members shot the little girl and injured two other passengers in the car. Had the driver not reacted very quickly, more slayings would have resulted.

Another recent report documented juvenile crime. Entitled "The Rise of the Young and the Ruthless," the article warned that America's children were turning to crime at such an alarming rate that juvenile arrests were likely to double by the year 2010. Juveniles were found to be responsible for one out of every five violent crimes. Between 1983 and 1992, violations of juvenile weapons more than doubled for each racial group. From 1983 to 1992, the number of gun-related murders of juveniles increased fivefold. The authors found that one quarter of juvenile victims were killed by other children. Finally, from 1980 to 1992, the number of children who were subjects of child abuse and neglect nearly tripled, from one million to almost three million children.[7]

Still another article reported that a thirteen-year-old girl, fascinated with horror, was convicted of smothering to death two young children in her care. She apparently loved anything that stood for Halloween: darkness, masks, and scaring little children.[8]

We find this violent, even murderous, trend in children to be tragic and an extremely disturbing reflection of the state of our society. Homeopathy, as you will see in the cases you are about to read, can turn many of these children around so that they do not turn into killers or victims.

These violent, even criminal, behaviors fall under the diagnostic category of Conduct Disorder, which is estimated to include 4 to 10 percent of children. The diagnosis is based on a violation of the basic rights of others and of age-appropriate societal norms.[9] "Conduct-disordered children exhibit a pattern of behavior that includes aggression, theft, vandalism, fire setting, opposition to authority, and other antisocial behaviors."[10] To be diagnosed with a conduct disorder, a child must have

[7] *Seattle Times,* September 11, 1995, p. A5.
[8] *Seattle Times* , November 3, 1995.
[9] Schroeder and Gordon, op. cit., 280.
[10] Ibid., 280.

done at least three of the following for at least six months: stealing, running away, lying, arson, truancy, breaking and entering, destroying property, cruelty to animals or people, forced sexual activity, using a weapon in fights, and initiating fights. Teachers, counselors, and other parents often complain about these youngsters hurting others or behaving unacceptably. In extreme cases, these children can be very frightening to parents and teachers.

"I'm Gonna Kill You!"

Peter was a bubbly, blond seven-year-old. His Mariners sweatshirt and baseball cap fit the bill of a Little Leaguer. Peter's mom described him as "neurologically disorganized." "He didn't come out settled at birth. He's always been oversensitive to light and noise. Peter's system just isn't in synch. He's under stress all the time. Anything can tip the scale for him." From birth, Peter cried constantly. His only solace came from being rocked.

A loud talker, Peter could experience severe mood and behavioral swings, like Jekyll and Hyde. He would be really sweet one minute and threaten "I'm gonna kill you" the next. He could either be really gentle with the family cat or haul it all from room to room. Peter was very easily frustrated. During his violent rages, he kicked, threw things, swore, and talked repeatedly of killing people. He would yell all the awful words he could think of at the time. He bashed his toys. When he was the maddest, Peter would yell, "I'm gonna get a gun and shoot you. I'll hit you. I hate you." When younger, Peter used to bite others. He had no self-restraint. When we first saw him, his rages occurred at least twice a month. When he was younger, they occurred several times a week.

This was only one side of Peter. The other side was sweet, intelligent, and didn't want to hurt anyone. Peter often lamented to his mother, "I'm really stupid, dumb. Help me stop doing this." But he could not stop himself. The child was also an incredible actor and singer and had a rich fantasy world.

Peter's concentration was "all over the map." He was up and down in his chair at school and frequently got into fights with other children. He was terrified of the dark and of dogs, and had been afraid to put his head under water. Peter had recurrent nightmares about monsters trying to get him, making him scream out in the middle of the night.

What struck us the most about Peter was the violence of all of his responses. Whether fearfulness or rage,

Stramonium
(*Datura stramonium* or thorn apple)

Children matching the picture of *Stramonium* exhibit a mixture of extreme fear and violence. The feeling is like the terror of being in a dark jungle surrounded by wild animals who may attack them at any moment, and the response is violence and rage. These children are very afraid of the dark, especially when alone, and can become extremely clingy. They may become violent if provoked. They fear animals, water, and violent death. They often have nightmares or terrors with shrieking. Stammering, cursing, jealousy, and rage are common behaviors. These are very intense children. A very frightening or traumatic event such as violent abuse or birth trauma may catapult a child into a *Stramonium* state.

Peter always responded to the world as if he were in immediate danger and needed to respond violently. This violence and the numerous fears, especially of dogs, monsters, and the water, are classic for the medicine *Stramonium*. This medicine can be particularly helpful for people who fly into such powerful episodes of rage that it seems like something beyond them takes over, making them wild out of all normal proportion. The eruption of anger in people needing this medicine seems to reflect unconscious, raw animal instincts. Those needing this medicine tend to feel as if they are alone in the forest surrounded by dangerous wild animals and must be on guard at every moment, particularly in the dark.

Peter's mother noticed the difference in him within three days after he took *Stramonium*. He was much sweeter. There were no more rages. He was very cooperative and helpful and seemed happier overall. Peter was more tenacious with his reading and more willing to push himself. He no longer talked about killing anyone. His anger was one-tenth of what it was before the homeopathy. He was still very sensitive to noise and used earplugs in the classroom.

Peter was overall much improved from the *Stramonium*. He did not mention anything whatsoever about killing anyone until one year later, at which time the medicine was given in a higher strength. He has needed a total of five doses of the medicine over two and a half years.

"He's Fascinated by Violence and Explosions"

We had treated Kevin for coughs and ear infections since he was two years old. He was always a kind, caring child. Then, at six, his personality seemed to undergo a drastic transformation. Suddenly, for no explicable reason, he developed a dark streak. He became fascinated by violence and explosions and began to be obsessed with the *Hindenburg* blowing up. His behavior seemed paradoxical. He laughed when others got hurt but consoled other children in the nurse's office. Kevin started to hit, swear, and kick. He appeared to be as angry with himself as with others. His parents were in disbelief about how much and how quickly Kevin's temperament seemed to change. He had even begun to lie and steal. The worse his behavior, the worse his self-esteem became. He felt so bad that he even talked of killing himself.

Kevin was very bright, but now his attention was all over the place, except when he was separated from his peers. He could not handle overstimulation and could not keep his hands and feet to himself. He was very disruptive in class, always talking to the other children to try to get their attention. The teachers commented that he could not seem to listen. He asked lots of questions in class and was curious about everything, even the most meticulous details.

The medicine that turned Kevin around, as in Peter's case, was *Stramonium*. Again we see the rage, the violence, and the Jekyll and Hyde aspect. Two and a half months later his parents were happy to report that he was doing great. His focus had been good and the feedback from his teachers was positive. His listening had improved. He was not hitting and kicking as much. The lying subsided. There was no more talk of killing himself. He still wanted the light on at night and still had some fear of dogs, also indicators for *Stramonium*. Within another six weeks both fears improved. He needed a total of three doses of the medicine over an eighteen-month period and has been back to his loving, curious self ever since.

Tommy Fought with All His Might
As if It Were Life and Death

Tommy was brought to us at eleven years old for a behavior disorder. In a neuropsychological evaluation two years prior, Tommy was found to function below grade level in math, reading, and written language. He was shown to have inconsistent memory and weakness in visual and auditory recall as well as difficulties with logical reasoning. Tommy's parents sought out homeopathic treatment because of his severe, assaultive tantrums. His outbursts had worsened after he was put on Imipramine for bedwetting. Ritalin improved his attention and eye contact, but had no significant impact on Tommy's tantrums. He was even hospitalized for one month in a children's psychiatric ward for evaluation.

At the time we first saw Tommy, his parents considered homeopathy their last resort prior to giving him up for institutionalization. Tommy talked like a Mafia hit man. During his fits of rage, he was mouthy and would hit his parents, sister, and grandmother. He fought with all his might, as if it were life and death. He broke windows and punched in doors. Prozac, which he was currently taking, curbed the violence slightly. Tommy threw whatever he could get his hands on. He demolished his classroom after his teacher gave him too much homework. As an infant, Tommy had a habit of biting other children who made him mad. Tommy's mother described his father, who also had problems with anger, as having "a foreboding intensity."

The first and second grades were traumatic for Tommy. He was extremely shy and frightened to say the wrong thing. He got into fights with the boys on his street. Teasing was the worst thing that could happen to Tommy. He slugged anyone who gave him a hard time.

He lied and stole from his brother, played with matches, took apart calculators, and loved to go off big jumps on his bike.

Tommy was afraid to be home alone and feared the dark. He was particularly impressed by *Jurassic Park* and other movies where "guys got eaten." He loved dogs and wanted a puppy. He hated cats. His cat attacked him, so he tortured the cat. He had a fascination with knives and brandished them menacingly. Tommy sliced open the stuffed animals that he hated. He became very defensive, to the point of "going ballistic," and vehemently denied responsibility for whatever he was accused of doing.

Tommy had a history of recurrent strep, ear infections, and bedwetting. He loved candy, diet soda, pizza, hamburgers, and chocolate.

We found Tommy to be extreme in the intensity of his rage. His mother was fearful that he could hurt or even kill someone during his violent episodes. Tommy needed a substance from nature that matched his animal nature and violent aggressiveness. His behaviors— defensiveness, biting, hitting, and striking—are typical of a desperate, raging animal.

We gave Tommy *Lyssin,* which is made from the saliva of a rabid dog. People needing this medicine go into uncontrollable rages, often with remorse afterward. This state often comes from a situation in which the individual is tormented, as with sexual abuse or excessive teasing, as happened with Tommy's peers. There is a strong tendency in people needing this medicine to experience violent impulses to cut things, people, or themselves with a knife. This explains the anger that Tommy vented on his stuffed animals, which in real life could not possibly hurt him. Fortunately these violent impulses were not vented on live people or animals in

Tommy's case, as they could have been. Had he not been treated with *Lyssin,* it is quite possible that he would have ended up in prison for some later violent crime like the children mentioned at the beginning of this chapter. Five weeks later, Tommy's parents reported an improvement. He still had a few assaults during which time he pulled his mother's hair and banged her head against a couch. Now he was sorry afterward and apologized. In coordination with his psychiatrist, Tommy gradually decreased his Prozac without any negative repercussions.

Two and a half months later Tommy was doing much better in school. He had behaved quite well at camp. He had not hit his mother in a long time. He no longer hit or swore as frequently. He still yelled in a shrill tone when frustrated and still feared being in his room alone, the dark, and being alone at night. Tommy now mentioned that he hated swimming and would not get in the pool. This was interesting to us since a fear of water is

Lyssin (rabies nosode)

The main feeling in those fitting the *Lyssin* state is torment followed by rage, like a dog who has been kicked and abused over and over and finally bites its master. This medicine may be useful in cases of child abuse, particularly sexual abuse. The *Lyssin* rage is followed rapidly by apologies. These children are among the most violent and difficult to handle. Sometimes there is a history of a dog bite or being scared by a dog. Fears are prominent with fear of water, dogs, and claustrophobia. There is often an impulse to cut oneself or others. These children may be aggravated by the sound or sight of running water. Bedwetting may be a problem.

also characteristic of people needing *Lyssin*. (Rabies is also called "hydrophobia".) Tommy still had a demanding nature and expected his mother to be his servant.

Six months after he was given *Lyssin,* Tommy's behavior continued to improve. He was no longer violent, and engaged in fewer confrontations. His swearing had diminished. There were no more knife incidents and he no longer pulled his mother's hair. He still became defensive often and hated being teased. Tommy was less likely to throw things if he became agitated.

Tommy's case is still in progress. Needless to say, he has a way to go but his behavior is now manageable. Tommy's mother does not live in fear of being seriously hurt or killed by him and his parents did not need to institutionalize him. Tommy will need to continue to receive homeopathic treatment for at least two more years.

"Everything He Does Is Too Intense"

Kirk's mother knew nothing about homeopathy, but she had read one of our articles about homeopathic treatment of ADD and was willing to try almost anything to civilize her son. Kirk, age seven, had tried all of the ADD medications, each of which caused side effects. The most recent one, an antidepressant, had resulted in blinking eyes, shoulder shrugs, and tics. Kirk's mother described him wearily: "He bugs people; he's in their face. He just can't settle down or concentrate. He moves at such a fast pace. It's irritating. In groups, he's always the bad guy. He can't wait for his turn. When he gets mad, he slugs and kicks. He's all-around obnoxious. Kirk's impulsive. He has to have everything right now. He even pulls out his loose teeth before they fall out. He never thinks about the consequences."

Kirk's mom home-schooled him, as is typical with many of the children in our practice. He found math easy but he still could not read. He had a hard time remembering what he learned.

Power and control were vital to Kirk. His family lived on a farm and he loved to chase the chickens and ride the calf. When he got mad, Kirk became very destructive. He hurled his toys and stomped on them. Kirk held grudges and was unforgiving of anyone who wronged him. He had absolutely no remorse when he hurt others. Tripping others was good sport.

Kirk's mother continued, "Everything he does is too intense. He runs over his baby sister without thinking. He hits his siblings then smirks and says they deserved it. Seeing others get into trouble is exciting to him. He pesters his brother and sisters and just won't quit." Kirk was "tender with a hard shell." His self-esteem was low. He felt that nobody loved him.

Kirk had been a perfect angel until he was three, when his sister was born. He would hold the baby by the neck. His mother feared that he would strangle his sister and would not let him carry her. Once he struck her. Another time he stuck his finger down her throat.

Terrified of the dark, Kirk needed to have his mother by his side at night. He hated loud noises and used to cry when he heard fireworks or the lawn mower. He had night terrors when he was younger.

Kirk still was not potty trained; he had never been dry at night and had some wet spots during the day. He also complained of headaches "like someone is really pounding my head."

We prescribed *Stramonium* for Kirk because of his violent tendencies. At his four-month follow-up, Kirk's mother described how he had improved in every area and that the tics, which remained from the antidepressant, were gone. "Now he's sensitive. He even picked a flower for me yesterday. Before he didn't even have a conscience. He trips other kids now only if they provoke him."

Kirk's behavior continued to improve on the *Stramonium*. He needed a dose of the medicine on an average of once every three months. Generally one dose of a homeopathic medicine lasts four to six months or longer.

Two and a half years after beginning treatment, Kirk's mother felt that the *Stramonium* was no longer working well. At this time she provided more details about her son's behavior when the homeopathic medicine was not working. His arguments with his sister began with verbal battering and lack of cooperation then escalated into kicking, punching, and hair-pulling. It was a matter of power and control.

What disturbed his mother the most about Kirk was his complete lack of compassion and remorse. When his baby sister got her finger slammed in the car door, he did not offer to help. Kirk and some other boys got into a rock-throwing fight at the church barbecue. When his rock hit another child in the eye, he seemed pleased and told his mom it was the other boy's fault.

Kirk's mom recounted to us for the first time his experience with beebees the year before. He shot a bird in the air, a goat in the udder, and the family's pet cat. He lied and told his parents their pet dog attacked the cat. When his father threatened to shoot the dog, Kirk still did not admit to what he had done. When they took the cat to the vet, they found the beebees. Kirk acted as if he had done nothing wrong.

Kirk's total lack of conscience was very striking. He was intentionally malicious toward others and when they were hurt he showed absolutely no remorse. We could only imagine where this would lead Kirk as an adult if his behavior remained unchecked. This type of meanness with a lack of any conscience led us to give Kirk a medicine for people who care little about others, isolate themselves, build up a store of tremendous anger, then strike out in a cruel, even inhuman way. They may even become so savagely rageful that they kill someone without regret. They lack the moral conscience that is the guiding principle for most members of society. This substance is *Scorpion.*

Three months after we prescribed *Scorpion* for Kirk, his mother reported a distinct improvement. Instead of hurting his siblings when he became angry, he would now walk away. He was helping them more and being more protective. He was no longer physically aggressive. Time-outs, which were previously futile, now worked

Scorpion (androctonos)

The scorpion lives under rocks in the desert and stings its prey to death by sudden attacks. Children who need *Scorpion* lack a conscience and compassion for the suffering of others. They can be extremely violent, hurting or even murdering others if provoked or just for the fun of it. Parents of these children often fear bodily harm or that their children are headed for a life of criminal violence. These children are detached from other people and like to be alone, removed from the demands of society, as though they are viewing the world distantly through a small hole in the rocks. They are absolutely self-centered. Indifferent to pleasure or pain, to others' opinion of them, and to any duties or responsibilities, they live in self-imposed isolation.

well with Kirk. His attention and attitude had also improved. Kirk's mother concluded, "He's nicer. We can live with him." He has needed intermittent repetitions of the *Scorpion*. When he relapses, he turns into a different person, one whom his mother despises, and she calls us immediately for help. Fortunately we treat Kirk's mother and siblings, which has made it somewhat easier for the whole family to cope with Kirk.

"Drew Hits, Kicks, Punches, Thrashes, Throws, and Screams"

Drew's photo showed a child with light blond hair, freckles, and big blue eyes with mischief pouring out of them. He had a great smile. We never met this child personally since we treated him by telephone consultation. His parents' biggest concern was Drew's temper. He had exhibited violent outbursts since the age of fourteen months. If he wanted to do something and his parents refused, Drew ran in circles. When he got mad, he picked up large metal toy trucks and threw them at the nearest person. When his parents told him "No, you can't," he responded by hitting, kicking, and punching them. If they tried to give him a time-out and send him to his room, he trashed it and threw his toys down the steps. At the age of two, Drew slammed the dining room chairs on the ground. He made a beeline to any objects that he knew his parents treasured. Whatever was close was fair game for destruction, including the family dog, whom Drew kicked if she was in his way. His parents had to remind him constantly to leave the dog alone. Once he was rushed to the emergency room and received stitches above his eye after he threw himself against a glass coffee table during one of his tantrums. His bewildered mother said it was like having two different children in one.

These fits lasted about half an hour. There was absolutely nothing Drew's parents could do to calm him down. If they approached to try to comfort him, the madder he became. He did not want to be touched or held when he was mad. But when he was finished tantrumming, he put out his arms, said he was sorry, and wanted to be held. When his mother tried to discuss these episodes with Drew, he covered his ears and would not listen. He never wanted to be corrected.

Drew's kindergarten teachers commented that they would love to have twenty more kids like him. They gave him glowing reports at all the parent-teacher conferences. He was very social and got along wonderfully with the other kids at school. When Drew went to his friends' houses to play, the other parents complimented his behavior. He was so good that they did not even know he was there. At home he was a terror and fought with his brother and sister. He sometimes broke their prized possessions as well, which did not make him Mr. Popular.

Drew had a history of several ear infections beginning at age four. Otherwise he was quite healthy except for some warts on the soles of his feet and his right thumb. He loved sweets and repeatedly insisted, "I need candy." When we asked if he liked bacon, his mother responded that he did. In fact, when she was cooking steaks a few nights before, he asked if steaks were like bacon. He drank constantly and recently preferred ice water.

We chose *Tuberculinum* for Drew because of his destructiveness, alternating personalities, meanness to his dog, and strong desire for bacon. It is unusual for a child to be so loving one moment and so rageful the next. He was an angel at school and a monster at home. Drew's history of ear infections confirmed the prescription. He responded very well to homeopathic treatment. Five weeks later, his mother told us that his destructive tantrums stopped. He would still stomp off and slam the door when he got mad, but he no longer trashed furniture and valued possessions. He kicked a few things and muttered to himself but no longer threw objects. He still did not like to be corrected, even gently. The warts on Drew's feet disappeared after he took the *Tuberculinum*. At the time of the phone follow-up, Drew was rifling through his parents' closet looking for Halloween candy.

Drew needed another dose of the medicine because of a partial relapse of his symptoms after he used a mentholated lip balm which can interfere with the action of the homeopathic medicine. Drew's parents estimate an 80 percent improvement in his behavior. Other people have told them that he seems like a different child. He still has trouble differentiating between playing with the dog and being mean. We expect this to change over time. The warts on his right thumb went away. At the time of the last telephone consultation, Drew's mother remarked that he had sprouted two inches in six weeks. He was eating his family "out of house and home." He was no longer as oversensitive to being corrected and reacted much better when he was told he could not do something. Now Drew is considerably more pleasant to be around.

"Rachel Becomes So Self-Destructive that She Mutilates Herself"

Rachel struck us as intense from the first moment she walked into our office. She had bright red (dyed) hair, a look-you-right-in-the-eyes gaze and a certain determination about her. She had recently been caught shoplifting. She habitually lied. Her behavior had been violent since she was very small. She became so self-destructive that she mutilated herself, scratched her face deeply, hit her head, and pulled out her hair "in gobs."

Rachel told us, "There are a lot of people who hate me. They're always calling me bad names, making fun of me, and saying that they hate me. I just hate it. Ever since I started going to school it's been like that. Everywhere I go there are people who hate me. They just say bad stuff. They call me a robber. They called me that the whole time on the bus. I try to ignore them."

Her mother elaborated. Rachel used to lash out at people verbally and create a major crisis. She screamed repeatedly in elementary school and would not calm down. She hit her mother when she felt her mother was reprimanding her. Kicking and punching were everyday responses for her. Sometimes Rachel pushed her mother just for talking too loudly. Rachel generally felt bad after her rages and apologized.

Rachel threatened to hurt herself with a knife a couple of months before we first saw her. When she felt very angry toward her mother, the more her mother talked to her, the more deeply she would scratch her own face. When Rachel hit hard, she often said, "I'm bad. I'm stupid. I shouldn't be alive." She picked up cats when they tried to run away. She bugged her little kitten to get a rise out of her. Rachel had a hard time concentrating. She became easily overwhelmed but could "go into another land where she didn't hear things."

We asked Rachel's mother about her pregnancy, since the state of the mother during pregnancy often provides valuable clues to the homeopath about the state of the child and about which medicine is needed. Rachel's parents argued continually during the pregnancy. Her father was emotionally violent and controlling. He frequently yelled and swore and would occasionally break and throw things. Long contractions during the pregnancy frightened Rachel's mother. She was given Demerol (meperidine) for the pain, and Rachel was delivered by suction extraction.

Rachel's mother described her as a "Buddha baby:" bald, happy, and interested in life. Her behavior changed when she was four years old and was molested by a five-year-old girl at her preschool. She would never say much about that experience to her mother except to say that the other little girl made her do things she did not want to do.

She was afraid of the dark when she was younger and still kept the night-light on in case she woke up disoriented in the middle of the night. She also feared big, vicious dogs and was afraid they would "jump out and bite" her head off. Her fear of dogs was exacerbated by the "cat-killing dogs" that would bark at her when she got off the school bus. When she was three, Rachel was bitten on the face by a dog after she teased him. When her mother thought more about when Rachel's behavior became violent, she realized it coincided with the dog bite.

Accident-prone, Rachel tripped on a regular basis, suffered "a bazillion" contusions and abrasions, broke her wrist in a bicycle accident, and broke her knuckle twice, once punching a wall and another time hitting another child. She pulled a tendon in her thumb a different time, twice experienced eraser burns, and had casts four or five times for various injuries.

She used to be terrified of vampires under her bed. She dreamed that vampires came in and bit everyone in her family. Then the vampires ran away and hid under her bed. She ultimately lost her fear after dreaming about little vampire bugs on skateboards. The dream made her laugh and the fear dissipated.

We treated Rachel with *Lyssin,* a medicine made from rabies, which we have already mentioned in this chapter. We prescribed it because of Rachel's fits of animal-like rage during which she scratched, screamed, cut, kicked, and lashed out. Her history of abuse and her feeling of being teased to the point of torment fit the picture of the medicine very well, as did her rage with quick repentance, her fear of dogs and vampires, and, last but not least, the fact that her violent behavior began soon after she was bitten in the face by a dog. Another contributing factor was the violent anger of her father and the arguments between her parents while she was in utero.

Five days after Rachel took the *Lyssin,* her mother wrote us a letter reporting quite a dramatic change in her daughter. She told us, "It's sort of like the Buddha infant delight in the world is returning along with a heightened ability to incorporate the rigors of the world as 'normal' experiences."

Rachel has continued to do remarkably well over the past nine months since we began treating her. Initially she had better conscious control over her outbursts, and her violent episodes became infrequent. She became less accident-prone almost immediately. Within three months, Rachel was having only little tantrums. The most violent she got was to throw and kick things. She now had friends, for whom she bought Christmas presents. She was having "a whole bunch of good, strange dreams" rather than her nightmares of the past, and her sleep was much improved. She was doing much better in school, getting all A's and B's except for a C+ in math. Her grades just preceding homeopathic treatment included an F in physical education and a D in math. There was no more shoplifting or face scratching. She still occasionally felt the urge to hurt herself, but now she hit herself with something soft instead of cutting herself.

At her most recent office visit, nine months after starting homeopathy, Rachel was doing wonderfully. She had experienced no angry outbursts. She had not broken anything in a long time, or even thrown or kicked anything. She no longer hit herself. Her grades continued to be very good. She had just learned that she would be transferred out of a special-needs classroom into a regular classroom in the fall. She felt much better about herself, had no significant violent outbursts, and was no longer accident-prone.

As we wrote up Rachel's case for our book, we were struck by her mother's description of the change in her daughter after being on the medicine for one week. She used the word "delightful." That is the same word that had come into our minds in describing our interactions with Rachel now. She really is a delight.

The Eight-Headed Madman

Regan, fourteen years old, had been a problem child since the age of two. His mother was hospitalized for three months prior to his birth because her water had broken. She was miserable with morning sickness during the entire pregnancy. As a young child, Regan never walked but sprinted. He hit, kicked, spat, and jumped at a very early age. His father was also hyperactive.

The child was bright with a good sense of humor and a heart of gold, but he was a real troublemaker. He laughed over his constantly impulsive behavior. He clowned, laughed, fiddled, and chewed gum in his classroom. Regan dismantled his school counselor's typewriter, for which he had to wash dishes. He loved to be the center of attention. Regan often got into trouble with his dad because of his lying.

Regan was very unhappy with himself. He tried to overdose on pills following an argument with his parents. During that argument Regan smashed his stereo speakers and pulled out his hair. When he flew into a rage, Regan "became eight-headed and didn't know what he was doing." Following a hospitalization on a children's psychiatric ward, Regan was given an antipsychotic medication along with two tranquilizers. Previously he had taken Ritalin for a year and a half along with Cylert and two antidepressants. He still had significant behavioral problems.

Regan had an ordinary side, too. He described himself as "a regular kid on the move." He liked to ride his bike fast, to climb, and to build and deconstruct things. In fact, he had taken apart fifteen bikes. He enjoyed seeing his friends and meeting girls. He especially loved rap music; he found it so relaxing that it could put him to sleep. Regan had a preference for gang movies.

We treated Regan with *Tarentula*. At his follow-up visit after four months of treatment, he and his mother reported that his sleep was more restful and that, overall, he felt much more relaxed. Feeling calmer resulted in Regan's being able to concentrate much better at school. His grades improved from F's to A's, B's, and C's. Regan's handwriting was now quite legible. He had very few problems in class and no more suspensions, which had not been mentioned initially. The fidgeting and nervousness had decreased markedly. His sleep had also improved. In coordination with his psychiatrist, the family had eliminated the antipsychotic medication and decreased his antidepressants.

Regan told us, "I've been fine. I'm doing my work and keeping my nose clean. I'm not listening to rap music so much. I haven't gotten mad at all. I'm not even lying."

21

"You Never Know What She's Up To"
Sneaky, Mischievous Kids

Many of us read the comic strip "Dennis the Menace" growing up. Dennis' contemporary counterpart, who mischievously traverses the pages of this book, is Calvin. Sneaky children are at their best engaging, entertaining, and humorous. When carried to an extreme, however, mischievousness can drive a parent to desperation. Teasing and hiding can be carried to dangerous extremes. Lying and stealing may follow. What began as good-hearted play can turn into harmful, destructive, or even criminal behavior. All of the children whose cases we share in this chapter are good-natured, but all engage in inappropriate behaviors.

"He Acts First and Thinks Later"

Fourteen-year-old Phil was a likable, engaging young man. His mother's main complaints were that he acted first and thought later, and was erratic and compulsive. "He does crazy things. He likes to spotlight. He can be in the middle of dribbling in a basketball game and he'll stop and do a little dance with the ball. He's a very funny kid, like one of the Marx brothers. He cracks me up. He totally dismantled a karate class of fifty kids with his antics. The teacher completely lost control of the class because everyone was doubled over laughing." Phil had a dramatic streak. Despite a stammer, he tended to talk too loudly and be excessively exuberant. He was good at playing piano, but he only enjoyed music with a fast rhythm and pace.

Phil had his tricky side. He had a habit of lying compulsively. While his parents slept, he would raid the refrigerator and then deny it later. His hands could be full of ice cream and sticky buns and he would play Mr. Innocent. He took magazines, baseball cards, and other special possessions from his brother's room without batting an eyelid. Ever a manipulator, Phil had a habit of pushing as far as he could. He did not like to be teased and had a low threshold for adversity. When he lost his temper, he swore, threw things, crashed around, and slammed doors.

He was universally liked and had an excellent sense of humor, but could not make friends easily. According to his mom, "Phil could charm a bird out of a tree." Phil was kind to animals and pets and was infinitely patient with the family dog. He was always the one who asked about his mom when she was sick. He sometimes asked for free toys for his sister.

Phil's mom was disgusted by his sloppy habits. He lounged in front of the television snacking. He threw orange peels behind the furniture. His mother was constantly discovering dirty socks, Popsicle sticks, candy wrappers, and various remains of snacks turned science projects. It was hard to get Phil to do anything helpful around the house. If she asked him to fold towels, he would stuff them under a couch cushion. It seemed to be a kind of extreme carelessness. Once Phil even flicked lighted matches and threw them on cars.

Phil was home-schooled. He was not great at math or penmanship, but was a whiz at Nintendo. He learned best by teaching himself. He was fascinated by UFOs, ghosts, and the Loch Ness monster. He was very frightened by spiders, especially very big ones, but loved reading about tarantulas.

At six, Phil was put on Ritalin without success. He was now on Cylert. Already an erratic sleeper, the Cylert often kept him up at night. Phil's excessiveness could include eating nine oranges in a row. He loved pizza.

You can see that Phil was a character, and a study in contradictions. He was lively yet lazy, kind and caring yet lied and stole, was humorous yet rageful. Phil loved to be the center of attention, was charming, and often cagey.

We prescribed *Tarentula* for Phil. In addition to his sneakiness, charming nature, tendency to lie, desire to entertain and get attention, he even mentioned his fear of and fascination with spiders.

The six-week follow-up indicated positive changes in Phil. His mother had noticed a big change in his attitude. He had discontinued the Cylert, gotten a part-time job, and made a new friend. He was sleeping more and longer. Phil felt calmer, not as angry and jittery. The lying improved, and the swearing or throwing things stopped. The stammering was also better and he no longer talked as loudly. He was not pushing his mother to the limits. When people teased Phil, he did not react as angrily as he used to. His mother described him as more even-keeled. He was still a slob around the house.

Nine weeks later Phil continued to do well. He was still calmer and not as belligerent. There were no more angry outbursts. He started volunteering at a local community center to help other kids play ball. He told us that he was now thinking differently about his actions and was not as sensitive when teased. He actually folded some towels instead of wadding them up.

Nine and a half months after the dose of *Tarentula,* we asked Phil's mother to assess his progress since he began homeopathic treatment. "It's a night-and-day difference from last year. He's a nicer guy to be around. He isn't as volatile. He doesn't fly off the handle and isn't as nervous. He now has four or five friends and is able to get along with his peers much better. They seem to genuinely like him. He rolls with the punches. The basketball coach complimented him on his playing."

He Loved to Play Tricks on His Teachers

Dennis was a ten-year-old handful. He was a very active, creative kid. He had a bent for comedy and loved to play tricks on his teachers. He enjoyed "scaring the heck out of little kids." Dennis was defiant, argumentative, and "chafed under rules." He was an expert at bucking authority. He was always getting into trouble at school, so his teacher asked him to keep a behavior diary. Dennis pushed the limits to the max. Living with him was like having to read the fine print on contracts every day. People who interacted with Dennis often felt "taken" by him.

A born ham, Dennis constantly sought attention. He loved to act and dance, and was always inventing new steps. He went to great efforts to stand out in a crowd. He loved mimicry and could talk a mile a minute. Dennis's mother remarked, "If electricity fails, just plug in Dennis." He had energy to burn. He played the cello. Classical music put him to sleep and rock kept him awake. Dennis also had a precocious interest in girls.

Dennis had a strong fear of heights and a milder fear of being chased by dogs. He had a dream of a little guy with spider arms. In his dream a huge boulder exploded and a spider with a red rear-end sat on top of the boulder.

Dennis had a history of bad ear and sinus infections, allergies, and asthmatic bronchitis. His mother hoped that homeopathy could help Dennis with his susceptibility to allergies as well as his behavioral problems.

You have probably noticed the many similarities between Phil and Dennis. They are both live wires and real charmers with a defiant streak. Perhaps Phil, being four years older, just had a little more time to elaborate his act. We also gave *Tarentula* to Dennis. The mischievous quality often found in those needing this medicine calls forth the image of Dennis the Menace. Notice that both Phil and Dennis liked to dance, which is typical of those needing this medicine.

Dennis became "less manic" after the *Tarentula*. Eight months after beginning homeopathy, Dennis won a citizenship award at school. He even chose to complete extra credit. A couple of months later he was on the safety patrol squad and was volunteering to help younger children. He mentioned being scared of bugs that "come and wrap you in cocoons and suck you dry" like a program he saw on television.

It has now been nineteen months since Dennis began homeopathy, and his behavior has continued to earn glowing reports. He still likes to make funny faces, be a comic, and do whatever he can to attract girls.

Luis Hid in the Bushes and His Babysitter Called the Police

Five-year-old Luis had sparkling eyes and a very mischievous grin, as if he had a big secret. He was referred to

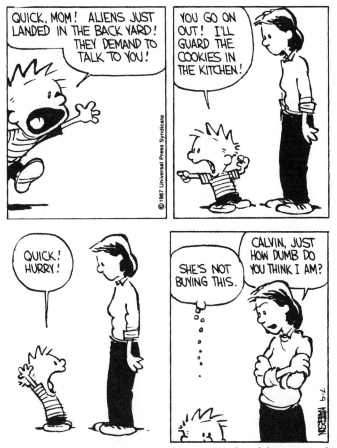

Calvin and Hobbes © (1987) Watterson. Distributed by Universal Press Syndicate. Reprinted with permission. All rights reserved.

us by his preschool teacher. He was very loving, but could be defiant and disruptive at school. Things set him off for no apparent reason. Luis was impulsive and curious, sometimes to the detriment of himself and others. When he went for class walks in the park, he would run out into the street defiantly. If he did not want to hold the hand of another child, as he was instructed to do, he would throw himself down on the sidewalk and have to be carried back to his preschool. His teacher was at the end of her rope, and he was on the verge of being asked to leave the school.

He loved to wander off and hide. He would disappear and not come when called, and he seemed to get a real rise out of teasing people this way. His mischievousness caused quite a problem for his babysitter one time when she could not find him. The frantic sitter called the police, and Luis popped up moments later from the bushes with a smirk. He also had quite a reputation for stealing sprinklers from the neighbors' yards, which was particularly unpopular during dry spells.

Luis' creativity and imagination were boundless. He wrote pages and pages of inventive stories. He drew a wonderful, intricate picture of a big spider. As he narrated the picture, Luis explained that when the spider died, it would feed the earth. He also loved to draw pictures of caterpillars.

Luis had a hard time sitting still during meals. He would pester his brother, tease, poke, and fidget. If he became bored at lunch, he would break plastic silverware and toss his food around. He loved to be the leader and tried to get other children to do what he wanted. When he got into a disagreement with his sister, he could hit, kick, and pinch. It was often hard to discipline Luis, because he cleverly sidestepped the consequences of his misdeeds with a hug or a kiss. He could also be sneaky about taking things from his brother's room and hiding them while pretending he knew nothing at all about it. When he was younger, he cut his clothes and hair, and said that someone else did it. He invented an elaborate story about a cat who cut his shorts.

Luis was afraid of monsters coming out of his closet and of shadows on the walls. During storms he would turn on all of the table lamps in his room. He was so sensitive to noises, such as vacuum cleaners, lawn mowers, and chain saws, that he sometimes wore earmuffs to dampen the sound. He was very loving with animals, except for spiders and bugs, which he liked to kill.

Luis was very cute, and just a bit too much of a tease for his own good. He was bright, clever, and almost too curious. His special attraction to spiders and bugs interested us. What was most striking about Luis was his desire to hide from other people, no matter what the consequences. Luis had the characteristic restlessness and desire to be the center of attention of *Tarentula,* but no particular love of lively music and dance. We chose for Luis another homeopathic medicine made from a spider, *Aranea ixabola,* a medicine which is specific for people who tease others excessively.

Luis' parents were new to homeopathy and did not know quite what to expect. They were increasingly pleased with the results. The improvement in Luis' attitude began one week after he started homeopathic treatment. The preschool teachers reported that he was more focused and noticeably less defiant, distractible, and disruptive. His mother found him to be happier and less angry. Instead of staying up late at night, he went to sleep more easily. The hiding stopped. Luis listened better. He did not hop up from the table as often during meals, and stuck with tasks longer. He had not hit, kicked, or thrown himself on the floor. During the follow-up interview, Luis talked about digging up worms.

Progress continued beautifully with Luis. He briefly needed a different homeopathic medicine, *Histaminum,* for his allergies. His spirit of exploration blossomed. With his father's help, he slid down the laundry chute at home. The only time he would lose control was when he was terribly hungry or tired. It has been a year since we first saw Luis and he is still doing very nicely.

PART FOUR

Homeopathic Treatment of Other Behavioral and Learning Problems

22

---cᴑ∞ᴑᴐ---

New Hope for Special Kids
Learning Difficulties and Developmental Delays

Approximately 800,000 children were classified as learning disabled in 1977. By 1986 this number had grown to 1.9 million. This is a different category from developmentally disabled children, whose numbers decreased over the same period of time by nearly 300,000, and the severely impaired group, which decreased by nearly 60,000. As of 1992 approximately 11 percent of all children enrolled in public schools received special education services.[1]

This chapter includes both learning disabled and severely impaired children, since we have found children who are significantly developmentally delayed as well as children who are simply slow learners to benefit from homeopathic treatment. Our expectations as homeopathic physicians are, of course, different depending on the individual child. Children who are developmentally disabled, with or without behavioral problems, can sometimes achieve amazing strides in behavior, coping

---

[1] Sylvia Farnham-Diggory, *The Learning-Disabled Child* (Cambridge: Harvard University Press, 1992), 10, 12.

skills, and learning abilities. They continue to be substantially more limited in their capabilities than other children, unless the initial diagnosis was incorrect.

We have seen many children in learning-disabled school programs who are very bright. They may have poor self-confidence, inadequate learning styles, or a family history of abuse or neglect with an absence of encouragement and belief in themselves. They may be dyslexic, have auditory or visual problems, have no inspiring role models, have physiologic sequelae of their mother's drug or alcohol abuse in utero, or simply be bored.

Each child has his own story to tell if we only take the time to listen. A youngster may need a different teacher, a new school, or may do much better learning at home. She may benefit from a radically different instructional approach designed to her individual learning style. Many of these children make tremendous strides after homeopathic treatment.

The Boy Who Could Not Stop Kissing

Jerry, a seventeen year old with a significant developmental disability, was tall, blond, well built, and had a very sweet, childlike expression and affect. He smiled most of the time. We noticed, on his first visit five and a half years ago, that he had no eyebrows. His mother explained that he had just shaved them off. Jerry crawled and sat at nine months and walked at two and a half years. At the age of three he was diagnosed with mid-range mental retardation and an IQ of 50. No genetic etiology was found.

As long as his mother could remember, Jerry had problems with coordination and depth perception. He suffered from seizures from ages three to thirteen, for which he received anticonvulsant medications. Jerry had a very short attention span and was unable to maintain eye contact. His hands were always busy, and he was always grabbing one thing or another. From infancy he only took five-minute naps, and slept five to six hours a night. By age ten Jerry was so hyperactive that his mother could not find a babysitter who could cope with his activity level.

Jerry was in a special education high school which would result in career training and job placement. He could only sit still for one hour at a time. Generally happy all the time, he loved to tease others. He grabbed people's wrists and liked to hug and kiss them. He even hugged and kissed inanimate objects like escalator rails and trucks. He was still uncoordinated. He had recently dived into a swimming pool for the first time.

Although Jerry had a delightful, playful temperament, others often found him overwhelming and playfully aggressive. His teachers reported that he picked on weak kids and harassed them. He enjoyed being the center of attention. He played with light switches and fire alarms.

Very limited verbally, Jerry often communicated through pantomime. His verbal skills were limited to "ma ma," "da da," "truck," and other simple, monosyllabic words. He was unable to enunciate clearly, so most of his words sounded the same. He easily forgot whatever he learned.

Jerry's judgment was poor. If his mother did not watch him closely, he would wander off. He did so a year before we met him and was hit by a car, resulting in two fractures of the left foot. He would use half a roll of toilet paper or none at all. If left alone, he did mischievous things like putting antifreeze in the crankcase.

He was shy when meeting new people. As a child he would walk around with a towel over his head if there were guests. Jerry loved animals but did not know how to be gentle with them. He picked up cats by the neck, though he never meant to hurt them. He rarely showed anger and was afraid of his stepfather's temper. He never cried much. Jerry needed lots of reassurance.

He had very few physical complaints, just some facial acne and a tendency to stiff joints. Jerry loved sweets.

Many of Jerry's characteristics are very typical of developmentally disabled people. Homeopathy always looks for what is unique and atypical about an individual. Jerry's constant busyness and his impulse to hug and kiss everyone were outstanding to us. We prescribed *Veratrum album* for Jerry. People needing this medicine, in addition to being constantly busy and hurried as mentioned previously, can have the specific symptom of wanting to touch and kiss everything. Jill, mentioned earlier, was an adult with a high degree of impulse control and was able to restrain herself from acting on her impulses in order to be socially acceptable. Jerry, who was unable to control his impulses, kissed with abandon.

As with many of the other patients we have presented, Jerry took only one dose of the *Veratrum*. His mother brought him back to our office four months later. She reported that he acted out more for a while after taking the medicine, then his behavior improved dramatically. He no longer kissed inappropriately. His attention span was longer, his eye contact improved, and his judgment better. He had recently spent a whole day moving a wood pile, which he never would have been able to do before. His listening had gotten a lot better and so was his coordination. Jerry noticed recently that he was dropping something and caught it before it hit the floor, which was extremely unusual for him. His reactions were quicker now and he was better able to catch balls. Before the homeopathy, he would throw the ball up on the roof and start laughing. Now he threw and caught it very well. He also kicked the ball appropriately, which was a new behavior. He enjoyed playing with the ball so much that he wanted to do it all day.

Jerry was attending better to tasks. He was putting away all of his clothes instead of stopping in the middle. The teachers reported that he was much better about refraining from touching others. The day camp counselor said his behavior was much better than the year before. Jerry's mother noticed that he was trying to talk more. He had begun to sing in front of others, even the whole neighborhood. He was now trying to put endings on words. He retained information better and his enunciation had even improved a bit. He had taken cooking classes for years but only since the medicine did he start to prepare his mother's breakfast. He could now make French toast appropriately, although he still needed help to turn the burner to the right temperature. Jerry has needed only five repetitions of the *Veratrum* over the past five and a half years.

It Took Todd Two Hours to Decide Which Toy He Wanted

Todd had bright red hair, a full face, red cheeks, and was considerably overweight for a nine year old. He was developmentally delayed and in a special education class. His mother was also developmentally disabled. Todd's father was unknown. He had an older brother of normal intelligence and a developmentally delayed sister three years older who had the habit of biting and clawing Todd. He compensated by eating. Todd, who was now living with his mother's sister, had gone from 63 to 104 pounds in five months.

Todd was not good at participating in group activities with his peers. He took balls and toys away from other children and ignored them when they objected. He ignored reprimands of all kinds. He was very restless. His aunt did not like to take him to the store because he wandered off. He was too friendly with strangers.

It was extremely difficult for Todd to make decisions. If his aunt took him to the toy store, it took him two hours to decide what he wanted. He sometimes became violent without apparent provocation. Two weeks before we first saw him he slapped and hit the school bus driver. He frequently misunderstood what was said to him and sat unresponsively, not knowing what to do or how to follow instructions. His learning abilities were extremely impaired because he often seemed to have no idea what the teacher expected of him. Todd was unable to read.

Todd did not masturbate, but he would strip down, bare naked, in front of others. He did not care about his appearance and often walked around with several inches of his bottom exposed. He scratched his genitals in public without any embarrassment.

Todd's chief physical complaint was a micropenis. His genitals were not fully formed at birth. He had been treated with testosterone injections at ages three and four without success. It was hard for him to stand and urinate because his penis was too small to hold comfortably, though the urine came out adequately. His testicles were also small since birth, and he had surgery for undescended testicles at age three. Todd had an obvious speech impediment, particularly when he pronounced the letter *S*. His cheeks flushed easily and he did not have much stamina. He preferred to take elevators rather than walk up stairs. His feet got hot easily.

Todd's main psychological and behavioral problems were his apparent lack of intelligence, inability to grasp basic instructions, and lack of awareness of his impact on others. We originally gave Todd a dose of *Baryta carbonica* (Barium carbonate) with no effect. When a medicine is given that does not best match the symptoms of the individual, there is usually no response whatsoever.

After restudying Todd's case, we realized that what was most unusual about Todd was the combination of his limited intellectual capabilities and his shamelessness about being naked in public. We prescribed *Bufo* (toad), a homeopathic medicine often prescribed for children with significant delay or limitations in learning, who may be much brighter than they appear. They seem dull and are often unable to grasp complex or sophisticated concepts. They may not function at grade level, but may be highly capable at one isolated skill or talent, such as an idiot savant. They may have the physical appearance of being stupid, sometimes with a protruding tongue. Often people needing *Bufo* have a shameless or inordinate fixation on sex and a propensity to frequent masturbation. The character James in the movie *To Die For* fits *Bufo* well. The young man was slow-witted and spent his evenings masturbating in front of porno videos. He was willing to do absolutely anything, even commit murder, to gratify himself sexually. Even when sentenced to life in prison, his sexual encounters continued in the form of dreams.

Two months after Todd took *Bufo,* his aunt called to say he was no longer having problems holding his penis during urination. His penis appeared to be an inch longer within six weeks after the medicine. He had also lost a significant amount of weight. Todd's aunt took him to a urologist who confirmed the increase in penis size and told her it could not be fully explained by the weight loss. Todd's cheeks were no longer flushed. We

Bufo rana (toad)

The poisonous sweat from a toad is used in homeopathy as a medicine for slow, coarse children with a particularly strong interest in sex and masturbation. These children do not comprehend very well. They often have a dull look on their faces as well as thick lips, which they lap with their tongue. They rely mainly on basic instincts and instant gratification. Music or bright objects are intolerable to them. They have a particular aversion to being misunderstood. Seizures are common.

last heard about Todd one year later. He had transferred into a regular first grade classroom and continued to do very well.

He's Off in His Own World

Shakur, five years old, sang and talked normally until he was two, at which time his mother used drugs, moved out of the house temporarily, and left him with his grandmother. Shakur's mother used cocaine, drank beer, and smoked cigarettes throughout the pregnancy. He was born after six months in utero and weighed one pound thirteen ounces. He suffered from chronic lung disease since birth and needed a respirator for the first three years of his life. Afterward he had taken a number of asthma medications. Even now, when he developed a severe cold, Shakur was put on a respirator to facilitate his breathing and prevent asthma. He was found to have a congenital heart murmur at two months of age and was hospitalized for nine months at that time.

We noticed that Shakur grimaced and made unintelligible sounds throughout the interview. One striking thing about this child was that he looked just like a little old man. His grandmother described him as very hyperactive with a short attention span. He moved all the time. Unable to communicate verbally, he was off in his own world whether or not other children were around. He preferred playing by himself and seemed unable to connect with other children. Shakur clapped his hands loudly, even in the middle of the night. When frustrated, he clapped even more violently. The clapping stopped shortly after his mother returned from a drug treatment center. He frequently jerked his head from side to side and sometimes jerked his whole upper torso convulsively. He made lots of spastic motions and gestures. The child shrieked loudly and cried fearfully whenever he was around a Nintendo game.

Shakur often screamed to get his mother's attention. He said "Hi" to his mother in the morning and stroked her face. Occasionally he even greeted her with "G'morning." The more excited he became, the more sounds he made. He was unable to control his behavior in an open area because he was all over the place. He frequently growled. He liked to roll in the dirt or grass or on thick carpets like a little puppy dog. He put his mouth on everything and loved to lick things. He liked loud noises like drums. Pain did not seem to bother Shakur; he never cried when he hurt himself. Shakur hated doctors and examinations.

Shakur's grandmother had no idea if homeopathic treatment could help him, but she knew another family we had treated and wanted to give it a try. She told us it was as if Shakur were stuck somewhere and she wanted to help him find his way out.

There were many aspects of Shakur's behavior and personality that were unique. He had come into the world as a crack baby and the genetic odds were not in his favor. Due to his low birth weight and premature birth, Shakur's lungs were not fully developed and continued to show weakness. His heart murmur indicated an inherent cardiovascular debility. In cases such as Shakur's, the homeopath does not expect a full recovery but a definite improvement. The extent of the improvement is up to the individual. Shakur's constant motion was notable, especially the spastic, jerking quality. So was his propensity for licking everything. His autistic-like tendencies, high pain threshold, and animal-like behaviors were also striking. The one word that sums up Shakur's state is convulsive. His every action, gesture, and word was expressed in a jerk or a spasm.

Zincum metallicum (zinc)

Children corresponding to the picture of this medicine are fidgety and restless; their nervous system is over-amped, with twitching, jerking, and even convulsions. The keynote symptom for this medicine is restless legs in bed. They complain a lot. They are sensitive, irritable, and can go into rages. With a persistent feeling of having committed a crime, they worry about being chased by the police. Their minds can be dull, with mistakes in speaking and writing. These children sometimes have a tendency to lick everything. They can look like little old people.

For this reason, we prescribed for him *Zincum metallicum* (zinc). It is an important homeopathic medicine for spastic, jerking, convulsive motions, and hyperactivity. People needing this medicine tend to have two unusual characteristics that we found in Shakur: the appearance of an old man and an impulse to lick objects, both animate and inanimate.

Shakur's grandmother did not bring him back to see us for four months. At that time she reported, and we readily noticed, that he had calmed down tremendously. He had begun to enunciate some words including "Momma" and even phrases like "What's up, daddy?" His teacher noticed that his attention span was longer.

Shakur could play with toys now. He had begun to interact with other children and was in his own world only 40 percent of the time now instead of 100 percent. He still screamed and licked everything. He had started to cry when in pain. Shakur still growled like an animal. He was no longer jerking his head, though he still exhibited some spastic motions. Even we were astounded by how much Shakur had changed.

During the ten months that we treated Shakur, he continued to improve. He stopped licking objects, was able to concentrate on watching cartoons for brief periods of time, and learned to play tag and basketball. His screaming diminished and his head jerking occurred only when he danced to rhythmic music. His vocabulary was still minimal. At this point we moved our office twenty minutes north of Seattle and Shakur's grandmother no longer brought him to see us despite our offer of continuing to treat him by telephone. We were very sad that he could no longer receive homeopathic treatment because he seemed to benefit dramatically. We are often asked if homeopathy can help crack babies and children born with fetal alcohol syndrome. Shakur's case gives us a glimpse of the possibilities of homeopathy with such challenged children.

A Case Misdiagnosed as Autism

Danny, a four-and-a-half-year-old boy with a delicate frame, was referred by the family practice physician to a psychiatrist who diagnosed him as autistic. His mother brought him to us in hopes of using natural therapies to treat her son. We noticed immediately Danny's tendency to scrunch up his face into an odd grimace.

His sleep problems had started just six months earlier. Danny woke up at night due to his fear of wind and the noise of cars on the highway. He awoke with agitation around midnight every night and again at four in the morning. He was also afraid of the dark because he might run into things. Danny would wake up crying and fearful, and make a mad dash into his parents' room. Lately noises had started to bother Danny during the day.

Danny was an only child and his parents had been married for sixteen years. He was a follower and somewhat shy, though he enjoyed being around other children. He talked up a storm at home. His mother described Danny as cautious. She could put a new food on his plate forever and he might never eat it.

Danny did not want to touch a plantain flower because he said it was too spiky. He was really sensitive to pain, whether little or big owwies. When someone touched his hair, he would scream. He was also very sensitive to bug and spider bites. He would develop big, open sores from the bites as did his mother.

His developmental milestones were normal except that Danny was slow learning to talk, but by two years three months he had learned the alphabet and numbers and was beginning to read. He was two years ahead of the other kids at preschool. He had always been very low on the height and weight charts.

Danny talked to himself frequently and often repeated to himself what his mother said or counted out loud in whispers. Danny found most cartoons too violent for his tastes. Danny had a history of molluscum contagiousum, a viral skin condition, and bedwetting.

Our first question was whether or not the diagnosis of autism was correct. The diagnostic criteria for autism include abnormal social relationships, a language disorder with impaired understanding and echolalia, rituals and compulsive phenomena, and impaired intellectual development. The syndrome, diagnosed by thirty months of age, is characterized by extreme aloneness (failure to cuddle, avoidance of eye contact), rituals, repetitive acts, speech and language disorder (varying from total muteness to delayed onset of speech to marked idiosyncratic use of language), and markedly uneven intellectual performance.

We did find Danny to be shy and not overly communicative. However, when he spoke to his mother, he verbalized well. He appeared to be very bright and curious about his surroundings. His mother reported that although he was shy, he did interact appropriately with other children. We did not feel the diagnosis of autism was accurate.

What seemed to us most unusual about Danny was his exaggerated sensitivity to noise. It was not that he was waking with night terrors or because he was afraid of being alone. It was the sound of the wind or cars on the highway that caused him to wake up, and then he would become agitated. He also struck us as being a particularly sensitive child, in fact oversensitive. He was sensitive to noise, to sights, even to new situations. These characteristics led us to give Danny *Theridion*, a medicine made from a small spider that inhabits the West Indies and is frequently found on orange trees. It is interesting to note that Danny and his mother shared the very strong reaction to bug and spider bites.

Danny's mother brought him back two and a half months later. He was now less anxious. His sleep had improved and he was waking more relaxed. Danny was no longer terrified. He was more enjoyable to be around and things did not set him off as easily as they had. He no longer grimaced or talked to himself as much. He still covered his ears on the ferry dock when the fog horn blew.

He continued to progress nicely over the next year and a half and no longer awoke during the night. The oversensitivity has not returned. Danny continues to function as a bright, lively, curious child with a shy streak. He no longer tends to grimace and talk to himself in a repetitive fashion, and he has not been labeled autistic again.

"The Parts Just Aren't Computing"

We are often asked if homeopathy can help children with attention and learning problems but who are not at all hyperactive. Ray was one of those children. He was not developmentally disabled, but, like many of the children that we see, experienced serious difficulties in learning. When he was twelve, Ray's mother brought him to see us because of his difficulties in school. He loved sports and he was very creative. Given a pencil or some Legos, he would go to town. Ray had an inventive mind. A couple of nights before his mother first brought him to see us, he had created an elaborate structure with a light, a hockey stick, and a number of other extraneous objects that turned his bedroom light on and off. But concerning school, it seemed hopeless. Ray would rather be outside playing.

His mother insisted that Ray was quite smart, but his grades were inconsistent. He got A's in art and physical education, a B in social studies, a C in math, and a D in English. Language was a real challenge for Ray. It was very difficult for him to comprehend verbal instructions. Understanding the meaning of words came quite hard for him. He just could not seem to form sentences. His mother told us that parts inside Ray's brain did not seem to be computing properly. This led Ray to feel constantly frustrated and enabled him to qualify for a learning disabilities program.

Ray had never been a very verbal child. He could entertain himself for hours and be quite contented. He tended to be quiet in social situations. He played with the neighbor kids, but seldom called anyone on the telephone, nor did he invite the other kids to his house. Ray hated to ask anyone a question or a favor. He was generally quiet in new situations, although he blended fine with other children.

In the classroom, Ray read at a fifth grade level, although he was a seventh grader. He sometimes answered a question aloud in class that had been asked half an hour earlier. Directions did not seem to come across correctly to Ray, even at home. He was often willing to do something and would begin to follow a direction. Then he would come back and ask, "What'd ya say?" He often lacked the foggiest idea of what he had been asked to do.

Homework was a real struggle for Ray. His mother had to sit down with him and prod him continually to finish it. She lamented that it was like pulling teeth, as if he were being tortured. It seemed painful for Ray to have to think and compute. Finding the main idea in a paragraph was beyond him. He could read a page in a book and have no idea what he had read. Ray would work extremely hard on an assignment, then forget to put his name at the top of the page. Most of this information was provided by Ray's mother. When we asked him questions, there would be a long pause, after which he consistently replied, "I don't know."

Ray was a concrete thinker and preferred to learn things hands-on. When his teacher asked the class what was the purpose of license plates on cars, he answered, "So police can catch robbers." He wanted very much to fit in, but reading and comprehension were a constant source of frustration. Stimulant medication had been prescribed for Ray, but made no noticeable difference in his abilities.

We gave Ray two medicines which had a partial response, *Baryta carbonica* (Barium carbonate) and *Helleborus* (Black hellebore), but they did not produce the kind of dramatic effect that we knew was possible. Homeopaths are like bloodhounds. As long as the patient continues with treatment, homeopaths stay on the trail doggedly until they find the medicine that produces profound, lasting changes.

Ray had improved somewhat from the time he began homeopathic treatment. It took us five months, however, to find the medicine that produced a deep, permanent change in him. This is longer than usual but can happen. We had focused on his difficulty with mental work, his problem with reading, the inordinately long time it took Ray to answer questions, and his contented state. We again thought long and hard about Ray. What seemed most curious about him was his inability to understand what he read. As his mother had told us, he could read a paragraph and have no idea what it said. This seemed very strange for a child who was inventive and happy overall. After restudying Ray's symptoms, we prescribed for him *Cornus circinatus,* a member of the dogwood family. Individuals needing this plant experience a disinclination to think, read, or work, and an inability to concentrate on thoughts. They read without appreciating the meaning of the words. That described Ray's problem aptly.

This medicine helped Ray much more dramatically than the previous ones. Those people who say that homeopathy is strictly a placebo should take note here. If a medicine is given that only partially matches a person's symptoms, no response or only a partial improvement will occur. When the medicine that most closely matches a person's symptoms is used, a profound effect ensues. Since he took the *Cornus circinatus,* Ray has done better than ever at school. His mother is thrilled, as are his teachers and counselor. His attitude at school is better and he is working harder. He scores higher on tests. It is easier for Ray to understand a lecture and to write a paper. When we asked Ray how he felt he had changed, he replied, "Everything just seems easy." He took the medicine nine months ago, needing only two doses, and has continued to improve in all areas of his schoolwork.

"Jake's Very Bright, but He's in a Special Education Class"

Jake was seven years old and lived in New Mexico. His parents found us from an article that we had written on

ADD in *Mothering* magazine. As with many of our patients, we treated Jake solely through telephone interviews. Jake's mother gave us the following information: "Jake was diagnosed with ADHD by four different physicians at age four. On a scale of one to ten regarding hyperactivity, he's a nine. He's very hyperactive, verbal, and boisterous. He's disobedient if he doesn't get his own way. He hits himself. Jake takes his fist and hits both sides of his head out of frustration. He yells, hollers, and becomes frustrated very easily. Then he'll scatter his Legos and flail his hands.

"He becomes extremely frustrated when he tries to do his schoolwork or he plays complicated block games. He's good at memorizing and is very bright, but he's in a special education class. He has one-on-one attention from the teacher. He's in first grade, but he tested at kindergarten level. Jake has trouble putting things on paper. He doesn't get his work done, doesn't pay attention, and becomes easily distracted. He's far behind; off there in the distance. Something's missing. He's not getting the whole instruction unless the teacher gives it step by step, one at a time. If you try to show him how to do something, all of a sudden he's looking at something else. Maybe he even asks you about something else. It's hard to get him to look and stay focused on one thing unless it's absolutely what he wants to do.

"He's been on Ritalin since he was four. Without it he bounces off the walls. He wouldn't even be able to look at his schoolwork. He's very rude and disobedient. I tell him to do something and he starts yelling at me. He's very disrespectful toward me. He's loud. He focuses a lot on guns and violence. He runs around saying he stabbed his brother.

"Jake has some obsessive-compulsive habits. He licks his lips a lot and sucks his thumb. At the same time that he puts his thumb is his mouth, he plugs off one side of his nose and starts blowing. He does it all the time.

"He's very attached to his stuffed animals. He has to sleep with them. He wants to take them in the car with him so they won't have to stay home alone. He wants to make sure that all the car doors are locked so that no one will steal them. He does the same thing with his toys.

"He's shy and keeps to himself. He likes to observe rather than to get involved with games. He's bashful until he gets to know you. He hasn't grown as much as he should. His brother is four and I'm constantly asked if they're twins because they're the same size. His brother is at the 95 percentile of height and weight. Jake is at 20 percent. They wear the same size clothes. Jake is the smallest in his class even though he eats and eats. He tells me 'I'm starving to death.' Last night he ate three chicken legs, two salads, and noodles. He eats more than me. He used to be afraid of the dark and had some nightmares. He'd wake up crying and screaming and didn't recognize me."

We asked Jake's mother about her pregnancy and labor. "I almost miscarried five times after the first trimester. My obstetrician told me I wouldn't be able to save the pregnancy. I switched doctors midterm. The second doctor put me on bedrest. I had Jake by Caesarean section one month early. He weighed under six pounds at birth and was very cold. I nursed him for six weeks, then lost my milk. He had ear infections starting at one year. The glands by his ears get swollen whenever he has a cold."

When we asked Jake's mother what she thought was most unique about her son, she replied that it was how much he ate and that he was very smart in his head but could not get it on paper. She told us that Jake's father was just like Jake when he was a child. Jake's father, like his son, was very active, was labeled as behind in school, was thin, perspired very easily, and was very, very busy. He always had to be doing something. Jake could not sit still and fidgeted continuously. Whatever Jake did, he did really fast.

We studied Jake's case carefully. What we found most unusual was the combination of Jake's shyness, failure to grow, difficulty staying focused, frustration when challenged by schoolwork, attachment to his stuffed animals, and swollen glands.

Jake benefited considerably from *Baryta iodatum* (barium iodide), which can help people who are irascible, hurried, restless, nervous, cannot concentrate, and have a canine appetite and swollen glands. It sounds like an odd combination of symptoms, but they were true of the medicine and true of Jake. That is a good match in homeopathy. If it weren't for Jake's restlessness and excessive appetite, we would have prescribed *Baryta carbonica*, a much more commonly used medicine.

Jake's mother called two weeks after we sent him the medicine to report that he had begun to listen better to her and to tie his shoes. One month later, she told us, "Jake's doing much better in school. He's concentrating better. He's down to five milligrams of Ritalin a day. Sometimes I forget to give it to him now, though he can still get somewhat out of control. He can sit and concentrate now and can tie his shoes. We went shopping for shoes for Jake. He started to get excited, then sat back down like I asked. His teachers have noticed that his concentration has improved. Jake's taking more time with his work and doing better. He's not as boisterous. He's not hitting himself as often. He hasn't had any dry spots on his lips from licking like he did before.

"His academics are improving greatly. Before they

had reduced his requirement to one new spelling word a week. Now he's asking for more. He's started to read. Before the medicine Jake was confused about whether one was smaller than five. Now he's counting to one hundred. Most of his papers are coming home completed. He started picking up hidden word puzzles since we gave him the medicine. He's begun to be able to put words in alphabetical order.

"Sucking his thumb is still a challenge. He's timid around dogs, but not as fearful in general. He's no longer worried about having to lock the car to protect his stuffed animals. He's started to grow. He was wearing a size five for the past year and a half and now he can't fit into his jeans. He's no longer saying, 'I'm starving to death.' He's not picking at his fingers as much.

"The pictures he's drawing are getting better. You can recognize now what it's supposed to be. He's writing

Baryta carbonica (barium carbonate)

The main theme for this mineral salt is dependence. The feeling in *Baryta carbonica* is being incapable of doing what is required for life without help. Those needing this medicine are usually passive and indecisive. Many children with developmental disabilities need this medicine. Their academic and social development are often delayed. These children may be slow to reach developmental milestones and find it difficult to grasp concepts or skills.

Baryta carbonica children hide behind their mothers and are timid about trying anything new. They lack self-confidence and like to keep things simple. They may also be delayed in physical maturity. These children are prone to chronic tonsillitis with huge tonsils. They often crave eggs.

much better. He's taking his time. He can concentrate now. The teacher wanted to know the name of what I gave him. It's a miracle. The principal said, 'You know, homeopathy's been around for hundreds of years. More people should use it.' "

Jake's mother discontinued treatment for financial reasons, but tells us that she hopes to start again in the near future.

23

---cXo---

Parents on the Verge
of a Nervous Breakdown
Cross and Fussy Kids

We have heard a number of parents say that their children seemed to be born unhappy. From their first grimace or words, some kids seem ticked off. We hear about people that get up on the wrong side of the bed. Some children act as if they were born on the wrong side of the bed. This discontentment is generally expressed first in shrieking, wailing, or refusal to nurse or have diapers changed. Nothing seems to please them. They may point to a toy, but when the parent hands it to them, they throw it on the floor. Whether this attitude or irritability and fussiness starts at birth or later, it conveys to the parents and others that nothing can satisfy these children and can be a source of great frustration.

"The Only Time He Stops Crying Is When I Carry Him"

Brent could be called a homeopathic baby. His mother, Holly, had been infertile due to endometriosis for a number of years until homeopathic treatment. Not only did her pelvic and rectal discomfort and other symptoms improve with homeopathy, but Holly soon became pregnant, a phenomenon we sometimes see with our patients. She first brought Brent to see us when he was ten months old. She was seeking help for his recurrent middle ear infections and colds. The colds began during a trip to Connecticut at the age of four months. One month before we saw Brent, he had been treated with two different antibiotics for an ear infection. He was unresponsive to the first drug and the second caused a rash. Because Holly had had such good experience with homeopathy herself, she hoped Brent could be successfully treated as well.

Brent was born with a right-sided bronchial cleft cyst and was circumcised when he was one day old. His mother was still breast-feeding him four times a day when she first brought him to see us. His first ear infection occurred at nine months, immediately after his parents fed him cheese. He had received an HIB immunization the day before the infection began. Brent became extremely irritable and fussy during his ear infection. He wanted to be carried all the time or else he screamed. She had tried conventional medicine for this first ear infection because she lived an hour from our office. After her experience with antibiotics, she hoped that homeopathy could prevent future recurrences of ear problems.

Brent's overall temperament was extremely moody. When upset, he immediately cried loudly. Whatever his mother offered him as consolation, he refused. Sometimes he went into crying, screaming fits ten times a day. It started when he was just two months old and had become progressively worse. The only time he seemed happy was when his mother carried him. Brent was a very impatient baby. He did not like to be alone and cried when strangers came too close.

Brent fits the picture of *Chamomilla*, a very common medicine for fussy, contrary children with ear infections, particularly when they are teething. Children needing this medicine, like Brent, tend to be whiny, restless, and complaining and are very easily frustrated. They may scream and point to one toy. You give it to them and they throw it on the floor and continue shrieking. But pick them up and carry them across the room and they're all smiles. The only thing likely to console a child needing *Chamomilla* is to be rocked or carried. As they grow older, they can get quite feisty and appear to be always ready for a fight.

Holly dropped us a note one week later to report that Brent was doing much better. He was even more irritable for two days after taking the medicine, as often happens after the correct homeopathic medicine, then steadily improved. One month later she called to tell us, "I've gotten my baby back." His ears were fine, she was

Chamomilla (Anthemis nobilis)

This common herbal beverage, when potentized into a homeopathic medicine, can become a godsend for parents. Children matching the *Chamomilla* state are angry and irritable to the extreme. As though in extreme pain, as they sometimes are during teething or an ear infection, they cry, whine, and complain continuously. They do not seem to know what they want and reject whatever is offered, even after asking for it. Restless, they like to be carried or rocked all the time, which makes them feel better, but paradoxically they do not like to be touched. They tend to have intestinal colic and green diarrhea like chopped spinach.

now nursing him only twice a day, and his temperament continued to improve.

Brent continued to benefit from occasional doses of *Chamomilla,* then his mother forgot about homeopathy for a number of months and relied on her local pediatrician. When she brought Brent back at twenty-two months, what immediately struck us was his tough-guy look, almost as if this little child had a chip on his shoulder and thought that the world owed him a favor. Brent had experienced a couple more bouts with ear infections, for which his mother sought out conventional treatment. She felt that she had gotten "off the track" of treating him homeopathically because of a second pregnancy and now wanted him to get back on course.

Brent was now an older version of the screaming, tantrumming ten month old. He became irritable very easily and overreacted to everything. If another child touched him while they were playing, he whined and cried. If thwarted, he writhed on the floor and threw a fit. This happened up to seven times a day. His overall attitude was "don't mess with me." A couple of nights before this office visit, his mother had tried to get him to brush his teeth and he had "gone berserk."

Brent wanted to do everything his own way and was very obstinate. He cried from anger or frustration. When his parents tried to set limits, his outbursts were so out of proportion that they did not know how to handle him. He thrashed when angry, hated playing with puzzles because he had no patience, and did not want to be consoled. Now the only thing that stopped his crying was to get what he wanted or to sit in his rocking chair. This symptom of feeling better from rocking is another indication for *Chamomilla.* The medicine was repeated and Brent's temperament again normalized.

"She Wants Things Now!"

Bri had a history of recurrent ear infections and bronchitis. Her other physical complaints included loud teeth grinding at night during sleep, constipation, and a tendency to scratch her vaginal area and bottom and to pick her nose. We noticed that Bri spoke more loudly than most children. She appeared demonstrative, expressive, and lively during the interview. She had a sly grin on her face.

Her mom described Bri as impatient and sharp. Her nature was not as sweet as that of her younger sister. She wanted things immediately. She was a very active, curious child. Bri had been throwing tantrums for the past year. When she was upset, she whined, moaned, and complained. Bri was a bossy child. She always wanted to be the leader. She was notably willful and wanted to do only what she wanted to do or she became fussy. Bri had very strong ideas about things. She seemed to want everything that she saw, but nothing held her interest for very long.

Bri needed the same medicine as Ben, whose story appears in the chapter about oppositional behavior, *Cina* (Wormseed). After taking the medicine her teeth grinding, nose-picking, and bottom-scratching improved considerably. Her tantrums diminished and she moaned and complained much less. Her mother was very pleased with the change in Bri. She has needed a total of five doses of the medicine over the past two and a half years. The indication for more medicine has always been an increased meanness toward her sister, teeth grinding, and a tendency to pick her lips. Each time the medicine has been repeated, her symptoms have cleared up quickly.

"Freddie Can Be Really Aggressive with His Sister"

Four-year-old Freddie was very active. He was swinging his legs against the chair during most of his initial visit. He loved to run in circles very fast. His mother explained that he could be very nice, gentle, cuddly, and loving— or very angry. He became really aggressive with his older sister. He exploded into fits of rage that he could not seem to control. His behavior could be unpredictable. He screamed and thrashed around on the floor. During his tantrums, Freddie yelled that he hated his mother, did not love her, and that she did not love him either.

Freddie's rage was often triggered when he did not get his way. He always liked to be the fastest and the first and had to be at the front of every line. He loved to run in circles really fast. If Freddie wanted to play a game and it was time for the family to leave, or he wanted a dough-nut at a time when his mother did not feel it was appropriate, he screamed and screamed. He knew he was out of control but there seemed to be no way to bring him back to being reasonable.

Freddie was extremely impatient. If he were not the first to do something, he became upset, threw things or stomped off. This did not go over very well with his sis-ter nor with guests, who always had to play second fid-dle to Freddie. His sister generally catered to him and was willing to play *his* games. Even his mother gave in to his demands to avoid a major fit. The night before we first saw Freddie, his sister was not paying attention to him so he picked up a small bamboo rake and hit her in the back. That definitely got her attention . . . and that of her perturbed parents. He was usually more likely to be verbally than physically aggressive, although the latter was escalating as he grew older.

The first time Freddie's parents noticed that he had a bad temper was when he was one year old. He was unresponsive to his mother's cautions about crossing the street. He plunged forward and she chased him. This resulted repeatedly in battles of the will. He ran into a brick wall once, resulting in eleven stitches to his head. A similar episode occurred a year later when he crashed into a thermostat. The scenario repeated itself when he hit his head on the corner of a couch. He was always running into things full force.

When he was in good spirits, Freddie was a good listener. When he was not, his parents told him things three or four times and he insisted that he could not hear them. When his parents tried to explain to Freddie after he had done something wrong, he replied, "I don't want to hear about it."

Freddie always wanted to grow up fast. He competed with his sister, who was three years older than he, in everything. He constantly tried to skip over developmental stages to catch up with her. He loved playing with trucks and cars and drawing very detailed objects.

Freddie's only physical problems were dry, red patches of eczema on his lower legs and buttocks, and an allergic tendency to a runny nose and puffy eyes. He often produced bright green bowel movements.

He was very picky about his clothes. He never wanted to wear the T-shirts that his mother chose for him. She had learned to put out a couple of pants and three shirts and to let him choose. He refused to wear shirts with buttons. All the labels in his clothes had to be cut out. He was also fanatical about his jeans needing to cover the top of his boots.

The medicine that we gave to Freddie is the same medicine that is often needed by fast-lane adults with type A personalities. They want to be the first and the best and they become very angry when they are not. The medicine is *Nux vomica* (Quaker buttons). These people are often very sensitive, insistent, and demanding. They are well known for their impatience and fits of anger.

Freddie's parents were very pleased with the results. They reported six weeks later that he was generally more rational. They could talk him through situations much more easily. He had experienced only a couple of tantrums. He still teased, but no longer to the point of defiance. He was still stubborn, but they could reason with him. He did not throw any more fits about getting in the car when it was time to go somewhere.

He was competitive, but he did not have to be first anymore or win all the time. He did not order his sister around as much. Their major conflicts had diminished considerably. Freddie had no more bright green stools. He was not biting his nails at much. One day he remarked, out of the blue, that he was going to stop. His eczema was no longer noticeable.

Nux vomica (Quaker buttons)

Derived from a plant containing strychnine, this homeopathic medicine is commonly used for children with extreme tension. They are hard-driving and competitive, and strive to be number one. These children tend to be hurried, impatient, irritable, and perfectionistic. They are particularly sensitive to light and noise. They have difficulty sleeping and often wake at 3 A.M. to think about things they have to do. Indigestion, constipation, and cramping are common physical problems. They crave fat, spicy food, and stimulants.

One of the most curious changes that Freddie's mother noticed from the homeopathic treatment was that he exhibited more feelings. Previously he had acted tough and never cried. Now he would show his feelings if he felt hurt, or would talk to her about it. We hope that catching Freddie's irritable tendencies this early in his young life will spare him and those around him from his later growing into an impatient, easily angered adult.

24

—⚬❈⚬—

"Nobody Likes Me"
Interpersonal Challenges

Every parent wants his child to be happy, "well adjusted," and socially accepted. This includes having friends come over to play, being invited to other children's houses, and feeling included in activities with other children, especially at school. It can be heartbreaking for a parent when his precious child is mercilessly teased by the other kids or when his child is always picked last to be on every team. A child laments, "Nobody likes me. Nobody at school wants to play with me. I must be a terrible person."

What can a parent do to help a child in such an unfortunate situation? Or what can a teacher do when he sees clearly that one particular child is being repeatedly scorned or left out? Or when a child is so overly sensitive that the least glance of reprimand or criticism results in humiliation and tears? Family psychotherapy, either with the school counselor or a private therapist, is often a helpful option, particularly when there are interpersonal difficulties in the family that need addressing. However, if the family dynamics are reasonably healthy, we have often found homeopathy to produce just the necessary shift in the child's outlook to turn the situation around in a very positive way.

"I Feel Like Someone Is Right Behind Me All the Time"

Natalie, age nine, could not keep up with the other children at school. She became easily distracted in a group setting and found it hard to concentrate. Natalie felt lost when the other children read too fast: "A long word struggles me." She did not want to admit that she was having a problem understanding what the teacher requested and became frustrated and angry.

Getting along with her peers was not easy for Natalie. They called her names and she made faces back at them. Natalie's facial tics made her frequently the butt of their jokes. Feeling hurt and resentful, she blamed the other kids for her troubles.

It felt to Natalie like someone was behind her, checking on her all the time. She even sensed someone following her during her sleep which caused her to wake frequently. This nervous feeling of being watched haunted Natalie night and day. "I feel I have to run because someone is chasing me." Only when her mother stood behind her or snuggled against her did Natalie feel safe. She was particularly disturbed by a game she had played in which Mary Worth was behind her and she had to stab her.

Natalie considered herself responsible whenever her parents argued. They had divorced when she was three years old. She had a tendency to reprimand other people. She described herself as a talker: "I talk about things that don't matter." Natalie was painfully aware that only she could change her behavior to get along better with the other kids but she did not know how to effect that change.

Natalie loved to bike, in-line skate, and draw. She hated smoking and would not tolerate it. She also had a strong aversion to guns, tobacco, and drinking. Natalie dreamed of horses and feared rattlesnakes because they could bite and poison her.

A warm-blooded child, Natalie's main physical problem was nosebleeds. They were quite severe, with clotted blood, and often lasted for fifteen minutes. Mild hives were also a recurrent complaint.

Natalie was the first child we had ever met with such a strong fear of someone behind her in her waking state as well as in her dreams. This is an example of a case where it was extremely important to understand the experience of the child. Unfortunately many children tell us that they do not remember their dreams and do not share their fears as openly as Natalie. Her forthright approach to telling us her symptoms made it easier to prescribe for her.

We gave Natalie *Crotalus cascavella* (Rattlesnake). Individuals who need snake remedies often have interpersonal difficulties. They feel betrayed, abused, or attacked by others and often retaliate in a venomous way. This is manifested in a subtle manner by Natalie's resent-

Crotalus cascavella (rattlesnake)

This medicine is made from rattlesnake venom. Children who need it feel that someone is behind them or hear footsteps following them. They have a characteristic fear of being alone and of ghosts and spirits and snakes. They can dream of hairy spiders. Intense, animated, hurried, restless, and talkative, they can suddenly strike out at others in a fit of rage. A characteristic physical symptom is hives, usually in one part of the body. Right-sided symptoms may be prominent.

ment of other children who "get me into trouble." Animals in the wild are constantly threatened by predators and environmental dangers, so they need to be on guard all the time. Natalie manifested this type of vigilance. She checked all the time to see if someone were behind her, and she was always nervous that someone was watching her. She needed her mother behind her to feel safe. She had trouble sleeping at night because she felt pursued. Natalie feared rattlesnakes "because they can bite and poison you." People who need homeopathic rattlesnake can strike when threatened, often in a violent manner.

Natalie reported at her six week follow-up visit, "The medicine really worked. I'm not calling people names. I'm not reacting. I'm not nervous." She no longer felt that someone was behind her and was now sleeping peacefully. Her reading, behavior in school, and overall performance had improved noticeably. Natalie's teachers were happy to report that she was more cooperative with her classmates and seemed eager to put her best foot forward. She had an increased desire to make friends. Her nosebleeds, cold sores, and hives were all gone.

When Natalie returned two months later, her physical complaints still had not returned. She had fewer problems at school. The feeling that someone was behind her had recently returned. She had a dream of a sea witch who was trying to take her brother away from their mother. In the dream, her mother had a glass of poison which she threw on the witch. Then her brother turned into a sea witch, too. The first witch had a potion that would make people die if it touched their hair. Natalie saved her mother and brother and the dream ended. The theme of poison even surfaced unconsciously in Natalie's dreams. We gave her another dose of the *Crotalus casavella* because of the recurrent feeling of someone behind her.

At her visit seven months after the original dose of the medicine, Natalie was having no problems with the other children at school. She no longer worried that someone was behind her. Her mother described her as "a lot softer." School had not been a struggle since she began homeopathic treatment. She was still much more cooperative, and her dreams were no longer frightening Now, ten months after beginning homeopathy, Natalie is still doing well.

"Everybody Hates Me!"

Belinda, six years old, was not happy with life. The family lived in Colorado and we had already successfully treated her brother by telephone consultation for his terrible temper. Belinda's mom hoped that we could help turn her daughter's life around for the better as well.

Belinda's mother described her as "a wilted flower." She used to be fun and cute, but her personality had shifted dramatically. She became upset at the drop of a hat and threatened to run away or kill herself. She expressed the wish that she had never been born. Belinda constantly complained that everyone hated her. She idolized her older sister, Mandy, who often mistreated her. When Mandy insisted on having her own bedroom instead of sharing, Belinda made a bed for herself in the closet.

Belinda's mother described her as inhibited. She was always afraid that people would laugh at her. She was too embarrassed to try out for cheerleading for fear she would not do it right the first time. Belinda was crazy about gymnastics, but, if the teacher ever corrected her, she decided she did not like that teacher anymore. Belinda hated to do anything wrong. If someone corrected her, she put her fingers in her mouth and wilted. She cried when accused of something or if her feelings were hurt, which happened on a regular basis. If someone rejected her or her mother reprimanded her, Belinda would announce that she wanted to kill herself.

She was clumsy and accident-prone. Belinda would walk down the hall holding her baby brother and turn around so quickly that the baby's head would hit the wall. She felt remorseful afterward. She was uncouth and tactless. Belinda had no comprehension of what was wrong with asking the disabled girl next door why she walked so funny or telling people to their faces that they were too fat. She made disparaging comments to her brother then passed them off as "just a joke."

Belinda's mother described her as a "fire hydrant baby." She would spit up her formula and it would come out through her nose. She was really fun when she was little: sweet, bubbly, and happy. Belinda used to be very outgoing and compliment people. She could be "Miss Social Butterfly." Now her temperament was just the opposite.

Belinda was quite afraid of the dark. Bad dreams woke her up, especially nightmares about people hurting each other or about scary creatures and monsters. Scary television shows really terrified her. She wanted to be right next to her parents during thunderstorms.

What seemed most curious to us was Belinda's personality shift. She went from being outgoing, fun, and life-loving to being an unhappy, even miserable, child who often thought about not wanting to continue living. A homeopath always seeks to understand what happened during an individual's life at the time such a shift took place. Often the person or the parent misses the sequential connection until the homeopath probes for the causative factor or event.

Sure enough, Belinda's mother remembered one specific event that immediately preceded her personality shift. She had been on the playground when she was five years old and a little boy hit her in the head with a rock. Now she was six, and her mother had noticed the significant change one year before. Belinda shared with us, "I thought I was asleep when he threw the rock at me. I used to remember how to write numbers, but after he hit me I sometimes forgot. Since that boy hit me with the rock, my mind just stops and I can't think clearly. Since that happened, it sometimes comes into my mind not to do nice things to people. I was never snotty before. When people are mean to me, I think I'm just a pile of trash. When the rock hit me, my mind just changed. If my brother or sister say something mean to me, I tell them I'm just gonna kill myself. I don't like living here."

There is a particular group of homeopathic medicines that are very helpful after a head injury and one medicine that is most prominent for suicidal feelings after a head injury. It is *Natrum sulphuricum* (sodium sulphate), which also benefits people who feel scorned or criticized by friends or family members. Individuals

Natrum sulphuricum (sodium sulphate)

This is a useful medicine for depression or other complaints following head injuries. The depression is primarily from being scorned in relationship situations or from existential anxiety. The child may feel very bad about himself, isolate himself, and may even consider suicide. The sadness is made worse with music. Children needing *Natrum sulphuricum* may be subdued or may have a wild side. They tend to experiment with drugs as teenagers. Physical characteristics include asthma and warts.

needing this medicine are highly sensitive and can become very reclusive and despondent when they feel hurt or rejected. They take insults or perceived criticism so deeply to heart that they may even feel life is not worth living. Belinda became so down on herself that she considered herself "trash" and became convinced that everyone hated her. It is shocking that a person can go from being so happy and outgoing to so depressed. We have often seen this occur following head injuries. We were relieved to hear from Belinda's mother five weeks later that she was doing much better. She was considerably less accident-prone. Her ability to stay on task and concentrate was substantially improved. She was no longer mean, and had stopped talking about wanting to die. She was much less sensitive. Belinda reported, "I can remember stuff that I couldn't remember before like what I am going to do. My moods have been getting better. I haven't been getting very mad and I'm hardly ever crying anymore."

A call from her mother two months later revealed that Belinda was still improving. She was now able to act in a much more responsible way. She carried through on projects that she was not able to complete previously. She could stay on task without a chore list and follow directions without becoming sidetracked. Belinda was excited to tell her mother that she was making people laugh again like she used to do. Her mother described her now as "all-around pleasant." She was much more interested in learning and readily pursued her studies. She took teasing much less to heart and was no longer depressed. She made no mention of wanting to die. Belinda's mom remarked that there was a bounce in her step again and that her emotions had dramatically reversed since she started homeopathy one year earlier.

"I'm Weird. There's Something Wrong with Me"

Candy was a strong-willed child, but very sensible and sweet. She was seven years old and had many of the same feelings as Belinda. Normally very obedient at school, now she began to have problems listening to her teacher's instructions and had to be reminded about the rules. Candy's mother found this very uncharacteristic of her normally well-behaved child. Candy began to have a hard time following instructions at home, too. She told her mother that nobody liked her and she wished she were dead. "I'm feeling everyone around me is against me, even if they're my best friends. I can't trust people because they might hurt me. It makes me feel like no one really cares or likes me."

Her mother was also struck by Candy's outbursts of anger. "Sometimes I go to my room and slam the door or I get mad. Inside I feel so alone. I get all burned up. It feels like someone's hitting you or like you have a pizza party for your friends and no one shows up. The boys tease me and it really hurts . . . like you're falling and there's no one there to catch you. You fall flat on your face. It's like everyone's laughing at you and they're all your best friends. It makes me really sad. I feel like nobody likes me." Candy's teacher, on the other hand, told her mother that Candy had lots of friends at school.

Candy had a particularly upsetting time on Valentine's Day. She cried that she did not want to go to school and got in trouble that day, along with several other girls, for writing insulting valentines to several little boys. He mother had also found a family photograph with mustaches drawn over the faces. When she tried to talk with Candy about it, Candy replied, "Mom, I can't tell you." After much patience and listening on her mother's part, Candy finally told her that a boy at school had thrown dirt on her and called her a chicken. Most frightening to her was his threat to "mirtilize" her. She had even had dreams of running away from boys at school who were chasing her.

Over the next week, the situation at school deteriorated. Candy's mother got several frantic phone calls from school reporting that she was very upset and not getting along with her teachers. She felt sad and depressed and cried herself to sleep. She lamented to her mother, "My teacher doesn't like me and doesn't listen to me. My teacher told me that if I get another bad mark, then we'll need a parent conference. Mom, I'm a terrible person. Mommy, the sun's out and there's a big cloud in front of it. I just can't make the cloud go away." If homeopathy did not work quickly, Candy's mother planned to consult a child psychiatrist or psychologist.

Candy became progressively more defiant and would cry and cry if reprimanded, even for the smallest thing. She was adamant about not wanting to go to school. "I'm just gonna stay in bed and sleep. No one can hurt me if I stay asleep." She began to tell her parents that she hated them and would never speak to them again. When upset, Candy sobbed and threw her stuffed animals on the floor. She became much sassier and her parents were afraid to say anything to her for fear of an exaggerated response. Candy's only physical problem was a tendency to redness and itching around the vagina and anus.

What exactly was Candy's problem? Why was it so hard for her to get along with her teacher and the other children and even her loving parents? We felt that she suffered from extreme oversensitivity. She was very easily humiliated and the least reprimand caused her to feel that she was a very bad person. She was far too touchy and moody. We gave Candy *Colocynthis* (bitter cucumber), which is often needed by oversensitive, moody people. They become easily triggered by humiliation or hurt, and prefer solitude. They react with anger and indignation and can take everything the wrong way. It is typical for them to become defiant, pouty, and generally out of sorts.

We spoke by phone with Candy's mother six weeks later. She reported that Candy was able to handle herself without being too sensitive, and could take criticism much more easily. Her parents noticed a dramatic and positive shift in Candy's mood. Before she cried at the least problem and brooded for days. Now problems blew right over. Her red bottom was gone. She no longer had any problems at school. She was no longer defiant, but still strong-willed. Her mother explained, "She's gonna do what she's gonna do. She thinks she's grown up." We found this to be quite normal.

Candy has continued to derive great benefit from *Colocynthis* over the past two years since it was first given to her and has needed only two repetitions of the medicine.

Colocynthis (bitter cucumber)

Anger and indignation are the main feelings for people needing *Colocynthis*. These children are easily offended, especially by insults, humiliation, or feeling unappreciated. They are highly sensitive. Cramping pains, particularly in the abdomen, or sciatic pains in the legs are the most frequent physical problems. The pains are relieved by hard pressure or bending over.

25

"Life Is Like a Vacuum Cleaner. It Sucks."

Depressed Kids

We generally think of children as happy-go-lucky and excited about life. Some children, however, are often despondent and apathetic, can dislike, or even hate, themselves and their lives. We are not just speaking of children who come from a background of abuse of neglect. Some of these children come from loving, caring families. They may demonstrate their despair overtly or may hold it deep inside, appearing to be cheerful to those around them.

The prevalence of depression during childhood varies greatly according to research studies, ranging from 1.9 to 13.9 percent. Higher prevalence rates are found among children from special populations, such as children who are referred for learning problems.[2]

A recent story entitled "Japanese boy kills self over bullying" recounted this tragedy.[3] Leaving a farewell note explaining that classmates' bullying had made him

---

[2] Philip C. Kendall, ed., *Child and Adolescent Therapy. Cognitive-Behavioral Procedures* (New York: The Guilford Press, 1991), 171-2.
[3] *Seattle Times,* November 28, 1995.

scared to live, a thirteen-year-old boy from Tokyo became the latest victim of suicide in a highly conformist society. The boy wrote, in his suicide note, "They are bullying other classmates, too. I will sacrifice myself, as they don't know how bad bullying is." In the past year at least ten schoolboys in Japan have taken their own lives due to being teased, tormented, or ostracized by other children. It is fascinating to us, as homeopaths, that one of the primary medicines for suicidal depression, *Natrum sulphuricum*, is also given to people who are extremely sensitive to scorn. Perhaps some of these boys' lives could have been spared had they been treated homeopathically.

We have noticed, among contemporary teenagers in the United States, a particular trend toward nihilism, negativity, and pessimism. The following case is an example of that trend.

"I Feel Hateful and Vengeful, and Nobody Cares"

Brian's mother brought him for help when he was sixteen. At the time of his first appointment, Brian first denied having any problems. "Nothing at all is wrong. I don't have a life. I don't have freedom. I don't have anything. Life is like a vacuum cleaner. Even when it's really working, it sucks. I have no friends. There's nothing that I like to do and no one I can relate to." His mother felt that it was urgent for us to see him because, during a recent rage, he had tried to choke her.

Brian complained that his mother was controlling and blamed him for everything. He felt impulses to hurt her and other people. Brian sincerely doubted he would every be happy with his life. He found everything about his life depressing, worthless, and having no value. Brian's teachers complained that he did not pay attention, but when they called on him in class, he always knew the answers. His teachers commented that Brian worked far beneath his potential.

His mother described Brian as angry and depressed. He was judgmental of others and put up walls to keep them away. His harsh language and manner kept others at a distance. He was a very sensitive person. He used to be witty and happier and told a lot of jokes. But now he was miserable. It was as if he had an axe to grind against the world.

Brian revealed, "Most people hate me. I see no reason to love them. You get burned too many times. I quit trying a long time ago. I basically have nothing in common with the people I know. If I try to be nice, they treat me badly."

Brian fell on a sidewalk at age two and was once hit in the back of the head with a bottle. His parents divorced when he was four. He never found it easy to get along with other kids. He was always the one who got picked on. He still sometimes felt picked on and when he got really mad he verbally attacked the nearest person.

In third grade he threatened to throw himself in front of a car. In seventh grade he stood near a window and threatened to jump off the ledge. Brian reported having thought about committing suicide in junior high school. He felt trapped with nowhere to go.

We were very concerned about Brian. He was clearly depressed and very angry toward his mother. We gave her instructions to keep in close contact with us if there was any further violence. *Natrum sulphuricum* is the medicine we prescribed for Brian. It is the same medicine that we gave to Belinda in the preceding chapter. It can benefit many people who have a nihilistic attitude toward life and severe, even suicidal, depression. They have often experienced scorn or criticism from others and, because of their sensitivity, can build a wall of protection to prevent themselves from feeling vulnerable. These people often have some history of head injury.

We were happy to hear two months later that Brian was doing much better. He had experienced no more violent outbursts, though he still got angry and screamed sometimes. There were no more fights at school. Brian had stopped feeling that he wanted to hurt his mother or someone else. He still felt that people hated him and that nothing gave him pleasure. When we asked Brian whether he would like to not feel depressed, he replied that he did not think that was possible. Brian complained that his tennis game was not as good now that he was not so filled with anger. Brian's mother remarked that his humor was starting to come back.

Five months after starting homeopathic treatment, Brian was working half-time at a grocery store and saving his money to buy a motorcycle. He admitted feeling better, but was unwilling to attribute the change to homeopathy, which he considered "a complete rip-off." He seemed to have some investment in believing that something his mother found effective could not help him. Brian admitted that he had no more suicidal thoughts. Homeopathy has been quite helpful to Brian, even if he did not think so. Unfortunately, due in part to his underlying nihilism and his anger toward his mother, he decided to discontinue treatment against her wishes. They have begun family counseling which will hopefully continue to move Brian in a positive direction. We have seen several cases where teenagers, despite being helped by homeopathy, unfortunately abandon treatment.

"I Just Want to Die. I Don't Want to Talk About It"

Jeannie was ten. Her mother was a longtime patient of ours and knew that her daughter needed help. The family had moved from Seattle to Idaho a number of years previously. Jeannie's mother asked that we treat Jeannie by telephone, which we did. Jeannie was very pretty with blond hair and blue eyes, but she was not at all happy with the way she looked.

Recently Jeannie complained that she hated life. Nothing pleased her. She talked of wanting to die and of killing herself. She threatened, "I'm gonna kill myself. I'm gonna take a knife and kill myself." When her distraught mother tried to talk to Jeannie about it, she would refuse.

Jeannie refused to do anything her mother or teacher asked of her. She seemed angry all the time, dissatisfied, and very argumentative. If anyone opposed her wishes, she snapped back and quarreled with them. Jeannie's mom described her as a perfectionist. If it weren't just right, she wouldn't do it. Trying to make her bed without any wrinkles just about drove her crazy.

During fits of rage Jeannie would slam doors until the house shook, throw objects, hit, and scream, "I hate you. I want to leave." These episodes would come on very quickly. Even little disappointments threw her into a fury.

"I just don't like life," Jeannie told us. "It's everything. I don't like where we live. I don't like my teacher. I don't like our school." She did not like herself, felt jealous of her sister, and complained that her mother loved her sister more than her. Jeannie believed that she was unfairly treated all the time.

Jeannie had been very unhappy about the family's move to Idaho. She had a very hard time with friends. They were very important to her but hard to come by. They told her that she whined too much and was not a good sport. She was exceptionally sensitive and became easily offended at the smallest things. Jeannie snapped back at her friends, insisting that she did not want to have anything to do with them. She worried constantly that people would not like her, and when she was mean to them, they did not. Jeannie was very embarrassed by the warts on her knees and kept them covered with Band-Aids.

Homeopaths often notice a correlation between the mental and emotional state of the mother during pregnancy and the state of the child later in life. When we inquired about the mother's pregnancy, she informed us that her husband had left her during her pregnancy with Jeannie. She felt a lot of sadness. There was a profound feeling of being unsupported. During this time they lost their house and all their possessions.

Jeannie was afraid of aliens, monsters, the dark, dead people, heights, and graveyards. She feared the dark because she thought monsters lived there, and deep swimming pools because there might be a shark lurking below the surface or an octopus that could grab her. Once she got a frightening thought into her head, she could not get it out. Jeannie also feared heights and remained glued to her mother when they hiked along steep areas. Jeannie also had nightmares of people chasing her and trying to kill her.

When we asked Jeannie's mother when all the fears began, she remembered one time when she woke up during a fever screaming, "They're gonna come get me." It was like a craze went through her. She clung to her mother very tightly during the fever. She was afraid to turn around to see the monster.

Jeannie's only physical problems now were headaches, rashes around her neck, and an intolerance for hot weather.

We were struck by the intensity of Jeannie's anger and her fears. They had a violent quality. She struck out with anger unpredictably, almost like something took over her. As with Peter and Kevin in the chapter on violence and rage, we gave Jeannie one dose of *Stramonium*. It is also known as a medicine for fright following a fever or a traumatic event.

We talked to her mother by phone five weeks later. Jeannie was doing much better after the first ten days. She was more in control of her emotions, and now could even talk about her feelings, which previously had seemed impossible. She was considerably less angry, bored, and dissatisfied. She was no longer jealous of her sister. Jeannie had expressed no more urges to kill herself.

Her sensitivity to criticism and her self-image had improved, but she still did not believe she was pretty or intelligent. Her light-heartedness was beginning to return. The day before the follow-up interview, she told her mother that she felt happier than she had in a long time. She still was afraid of heights, but now she would go down to the basement, previously an impossible goal. She received the medicine nearly a year ago and has been just fine since.

26

---❀---

"Mommy, Don't Leave Me.
I'm Afraid"
Fearful Kids

Why Children Become Fearful

Youngsters become frightened for many different reasons, not all of which are apparent. Some children have a clearly traumatic event after which they remain scared or begin to have night terrors. This may be an event which they or their parents may be able to identify, such as a traumatic birth, the illness or death of a family member or pet, a particularly scary movie or incident, an episode of physical or sexual abuse, violence within the family, the birth of a sibling, or a particularly frightening experience at school. Sometimes the cause of the fear is not identified by the parents, but becomes evident during the course of the homeopathic interview. There are other times when the parents, and even the child, may never know what triggered the fearful reaction.

These fears can remain with people even as adults. One thirty-eight-year-old patient with ADD told us that she has been afraid of the dark ever since childhood and still is today. As a little girl, she ran as fast as she could from light switch to light switch to avoid the terrifying blackness. In her twenties she lay in bed at night frightened that evil spirits might surround her in the darkened room. Now she still finds the dark scary but, as a parent, has learned to cope with her fear.

S.A.D.: School Avoidance Disorder

Many children, such as Annie, whose story you will soon read, have an unrealistic and excessive fear of being separated from their parents, who are their major figures of attachment. S.A.D. (School Avoidance Disorder) is actually an official psychiatric diagnosis given to children with the following symptoms: unrealistic and persistent worry about harm to parents or fear of abandonment; unrealistic and persistent worry that a disaster will separate her from her parents; refusal to go to school or to leave the presence of her parent(s); reluctance to sleep away from home; avoidance of being alone, resulting in "clinging" or "shadowing" behavior; nightmares involving the theme of separation; physical complaints upon anticipation of separation from home or parents; and excessive distress when the parents leave.[4] Separation anxiety is normal for children six months to two or three years of age. When it occurs for at least two weeks between the ages of three and eighteen, the diagnosis can be made.

A variation on the theme of S.A.D. is School Refusal Behavior. Some of these children display an excessive,

---

[4] Andrew R. Eisen, Christopher A. Kearney, and Charles E. Schaefer, *Clinical Handbook of Anxiety Disorders in Children and Adolescents* (Northvale, NJ: Jason Aronson, 1995), 53.

irrational fear of some school-related stimulus or separation anxiety.[5] They may resist going to school for part of the day or refuse to go to school at all. This term refers to children who are anxious or fearful about school rather than children who refuse to attend school for other reasons.

Homeopathy: An Effective Answer for Many a Fearful Child

Conventional child psychology books attribute certain fears to certain ages of children. From birth to six months, for example, children are said to fear loud noises and lack of support. Fear of separation is said to come later, when the child is one to two years old. Two year olds are said to develop fears of imaginary creatures, burglars, and large approaching objects. At three, psychologists explain, children develop fears of animals, the dark, and being alone. Four-year-old youngsters are said to fear loud noises, such as fire engines, the dark, wild animals, and their parents' leaving at night. At five, more concrete fears arise, such as injury, falling, and dogs. At age six, they talk of fears of ghosts, witches, and someone under the bed as well as of natural disasters. More sophisticated fears arise from ages seven to ten, such as fears of failure and criticism, death, the unknown, and medical and dental procedures.[6]

Experts even go so far as to quantify the number of fears children experience. One study concluded that children ages two to six have an average of three fears and that 40 percent of children ages six to twelve have

[5] Ibid., 19.
[6] Schroeder, op. cit., 315.

as many as seven fears.[7] We wonder how adults would score!

This list and numerical assessment of fears are very interesting, but homeopaths emphasize each child's individual experience and select a corresponding medicine. If you ask your child to describe her fears or nightmares, you may be surprised at the candid response. During our interviews over the years, children have often revealed to us, in the presence of their parents, fears about which their parents had not a clue. A child's fears, whether or not the parent may find them logical or believable, can provide considerable insight into that child's state. Homeopathy can often alleviate fears and phobias, regardless of their origins. Whether the specific fear revolves around monsters, wild animals, germs, thunderstorms, bridges, dying, snakes, or impending danger, a homeopathic medicine usually corresponds to the state of the child as a whole, which can also help diminish the fears significantly.

The following three stories are about little girls who come from extremely safe, loving homes. These children are all home-schooled and are not subject to any dangers or threats from a school. These cases show that a child or adult can experience a deep feeling of danger even in the safest surroundings.

"She Gets Hysterical. She Claws Me to Hang On to Me"

Annie, six years old, had always wanted to sleep in her parents' bed. She slept well for the first two and a half months of her life and was a good nurser. Then her mother could no longer produce enough milk and put Annie on formula. She woke several times a night until she reached the age of five. She still wanted to sleep with her parents. Her mother tried to put her to sleep in her own bed. Annie told her she was afraid and would not go to sleep unless her mother lay down next to her until she fell asleep. Otherwise she would lay in bed and cry. She always woke up during the night and went into her parents' bed.

Annie's mom described her as high-strung and tense. She was very smart and caught on to things quickly. She formulated thoughts more like an adult than a child. Annie had a controlling personality. She gave her parents instructions, as if she were the adult and they were the kids, and expected her parents to do as they were told. Even when Annie was a baby, she was like a little adult in a child's body.

Annie's parents had been married for twenty-five years. She was very attached to her twenty-three-year-old sister. She always wanted her sister and her mom at home with her. Even when she went over to her sister's house she would call her mother all the time. She did not even want her mother to go to the neighborhood store without taking her along.

Annie's fear of being alone began when she had a virus four months earlier. The whole family contracted food poisoning, but Annie's case was the worst. She had experienced severe stomach cramps and vomiting. Ever since that time she was panicky that she would get food poisoning again. She told her mother that she did not want to go to school because her stomach might hurt (this was before her home-schooling began).

The child's fear about her health became so severe that she hated to leave her house and did not even want her parents to go out. She became frightened of going out in the car even with her mother there. She tried to jump out of the car twice because she wanted to go home. Sometimes, when Annie's mom went out and left her at home with her older sister, she had to rush back home because Annie would call her to say she was doubled over with abdominal pain. As soon as she knew her mother was on her way home, she felt fine. Whenever her mother tried to leave without her, Annie would become hysterical and claw at her mother in an attempt to hang on to her and prevent her from going anywhere. Lately Annie cried the whole time her mother was gone. She refused to go to school, so her mother decided to home-school her.

Annie's mother had experienced considerable emotional distress during her pregnancy. She had an older son at the time and, during the first few months of the pregnancy, felt trapped and afraid of having another child whose demands she needed to meet. She cried a lot during that time. The rest of the pregnancy went very well. Annie was delivered by Caesarean section because of her sideways presentation in the birth canal. She was put in a neonatal ward for nine hours after her birth due to respiratory problems. From the time her mother stopped nursing, Annie became restless. She continued to want a bottle "forever" (until she was four years old).

Annie was a very demanding child who nagged until she got her way. She always worried about when things were going to happen. Annie counted down the days before any event that she awaited.

She was extremely sloppy. Her room looked like a bomb struck five minutes after she cleaned it. Annie's mother had gone back to work full-time when Annie was four months old. Annie would be mad at her mother when she came home and clearly resented her for not being there. She had never been in a daycare situation. Recently Annie was very afraid of people breaking into her house. On a family vacation to Hawaii, some people appeared to be casing their condominium. This terrified Annie.

She developed occasional fevers up to 101°F, at which time she became delirious and saw witches with long nails. She was a very restless sleeper. She loved pizza, spaghetti, candy, nachos, and chocolate milk.

And so, the homeopath wonders, what is most unusual about Annie? Her fear of robbers? No. Anyone who had the experience Annie's family had in Hawaii might develop some apprehension about their house being robbed. Her sloppiness? No, this is fairly typical of children Annie's age.

We felt that what was most striking about Annie was her desperate fear of being alone and her exagger-

Arsenicum album (arsenic)

Restless and insecure, children fitting the picture of *Arsenicum* have a lot of anxiety about their health and often fear death, as someone feels who has been poisoned with arsenic. They can also exhibit great concern about germs and contamination and a disproportionate terror of being left alone. These children are more anxious and adult-like than a child should be at his or her age. They are needy, whiny, and impatient. Burning pains, asthma, diarrhea, and stomach aches are common in these children. Often freezing, they like the warmth of a stove, fire, or their favorite blankie. When thirsty, they often prefer to sip liquids throughout the day.

ated possessiveness of her mother arising from this terror. Annie's life was extremely limited by her belief that she would be in danger if her mother was not in her immediate proximity to protect her. This fear prevented her from feeling comfortable going to school or even spending the night at a friend's house.

We first saw Annie two and a half years ago. She has benefited a great deal from the homeopathic medicine *Arsenicum album,* derived from arsenic. People needing this medicine are anxious, fearful, and nervous. They fear that others are going to rob them and they have a deep insecurity about their safety and their ability to survive in the world. Individuals sometimes need this medicine if one of their parents has died or abandoned them, or even if they merely perceive abandonment, such as when Annie's mother went back to work. It is possible in Annie's case that this perceived aloneness in the world and fundamental feeling of danger and insecurity began in her first hours of life when she was taken away from her mother for nine hours because of her respiratory distress. This is not to say that Annie's mother should have done anything differently, but to show how early in life these beliefs and impressions can arise.

Five weeks after beginning homeopathic treatment, Annie's mother brought her back to see us and reported that she was much less clingy. Now she was able to stay with her older sister or with a baby-sitter. Her mother still called to check in every so often. Annie's mother now revealed that her daughter used to call for her even when she needed to go to the bathroom. When her mother answered, Annie would reply, "Just checking." Not anymore. She still wanted her mother to be present when she went to bed, but was now able to sleep next to her parents' bed instead of in it. She now slept through the night rather than waking up and crawling into bed with her mother. Annie would now go to the bathroom and for a drink of water alone at church, which had been impossible for her previously. She still preferred to be home-schooled, to which her mother agreed.

Annie went through another phase of being very afraid she would get sick. She became worried about germs and insisted that her mother boil the family water. This over-concern about health and germs is also common in people needing *Arsenicum*.

Two years later, Annie was doing much better. She no longer worried about getting sick and completely forgot about needing to drink boiled water. People did not make her feel nervous anymore. Annie's mother described her as much less high-strung and excitable. She felt fine in elevators and on bridges, which had made her uncomfortable in the past. Her mother told us that she had never remembered to tell us that Annie's concentration was also much improved after homeopathy. She also mentioned that Annie used to tackle her little nephew and even hit and punch him when she was upset. She now treated him much more gently.

"She Wants Me to Do Everything for Her"

At age four, Hayley was a very sweet little girl with beautiful platinum hair and blue eyes. She came from a very loving, tight-knit family of six. Her mother home-schooled all of the children. Hayley was "mommy's girl." Like Annie, Hayley was very clingy and cried for her mom to be with her. She usually slept through the night in a bed with an older sister, but still crawled into her parents' bed in the middle of the night about twice a week. Hayley insisted on lying across her mother's lap all the time. Even when she slept, she wanted to hold on to her mother or her sister. When she slept on her mother's lap, she even wrapped her arms around her mother's legs. When the family went to church on Sunday, Hayley did not want to go to the nursery with the other children. She only wanted to stay with her mother.

Hayley loved to wear dresses, especially if they were frilly and lacy. She loved to look pretty. She was quick to cry when she felt upset. Whenever she got hurt, she did not want anyone to comfort her except her mother, to whom she immediately came running. Hayley was a chatterbox. She was filled with a million questions. She expressed great frustration when she did not think others were listening to her or they tried to finish her sentences for her. She loved to tell other people what to do.

If her mom was around, Hayley wanted her to do everything for her. Otherwise she could be quite independent. She usually behaved very well, but when she did not, everyone in the house knew that she was unhappy. Hayley had been a fussy infant. Her mother had to carry her around to calm her, much more so than with her three siblings. It seemed to her mom that all she did for the first year or two of Hayley's life was hold her to keep her contented. She nursed until the age of two.

Hayley was quite healthy except for a history of recurrent middle ear infections resulting in surgery to implant ear tubes at the age of eighteen months. The only problem she had since was a thick nasal discharge when she got a cold. At these times she wanted, as always, to be on her mom's lap. Her mother, who had read about homeopathic acute prescribing, had given her *Pulsatilla* (Windflower) several times for these colds with good results. Hayley had been difficult to potty train and still wet the bed sometimes. She loved to take off her shoes and socks and to kick off the covers at night and to have cold air blowing on her. Hayley liked ice cream, cheese, and peanut butter and jelly and had an average level of thirst.

Distinguishing between Annie's and Hayley's cases will give you a good idea of how a homeopath makes fine distinctions between people. Annie and Hayley were both very dependent on their mothers and both wanted to be with their mothers all of the time, even in bed at night. But the two little girls' natures were different in other ways. Annie had a more intense and desperate nature. Her preoccupations went beyond fear of being alone without her mother and extended to fear of germs and robbers. She could strike out at her nephew when angry. Hayley had a sweeter, gentler disposition. Her only problem was her excessive clinginess. Hayley reminded us of yet another child whose mother described her daughter as "the Velcro kid," because she always wanted to be stuck to her mom. It was not even enough for Hayley to sit or lay on her mother's lap; she had to be wrapped around her. Loving as her mother was, it got to be just too much closeness. Hayley's dad,

Bismuthum subnitricum (bismuth)

This medicine is well-suited to children who cling desperately to their parent's hand out of terror of being alone. These children even follow the parent to the bathroom out of fear of being alone even for a few minutes. We have heard these children called "velcro kids." Solitude is unbearable. *Bismuth* is helpful for acute stomach pain in which even water is vomited as soon as it reaches the stomach. Individuals needing this medicine are often very thirsty for cold water.

who had cut the umbilical cord of her three older siblings, joked that the doctor who cut hers just did not have the knack.

As sometimes happens, the first medicine that we prescribed for Hayley, *Pulsatilla*, had only a partial effect on her clinginess. The typical response to a medicine that is not the best match for a person is only slight or none at all. We then restudied Hayley's case and prescribed for her a less common medicine, one known for its extreme clinginess. In fact the child does not want to let go of her mother's hand. The medicine is *Bismuth*. People needing this medicine find solitude unbearable.

Hayley responded so well to the *Bismuth* that her mother did not bring her back for a year, at which time her symptoms had recently returned after she had eaten devil's food cake flavored with espresso. She became more content to play by herself. Hayley no longer grilled her mother constantly about where she was going nor ran down the driveway of their house begging her not to leave. Nor did her mother have to give her three hugs and three kisses before Hayley would let her out of her sight. Hayley had stopped begging her mother to pick her up and carry her when big dogs were around. The bedwetting had also improved dramatically until the cake episode. We repeated the *Bismuth* for Hayley at that time. Her mother called one week later to say that Hayley's symptoms had already begun to improve again.

"My Most Fear Is of Being Kidnapped or a Fire"

Jillian, Hayley's ten-year-old sister, had fears of her own. She confided in us, "I get afraid at night. I've just lately been able to sleep in my own bed. My most fear is either one of us being kidnapped or a fire starting in our house. It happens every single night. I used to always go into my parents' room to sleep when I was really little. It was better until I was four and saw a television show about a fire." Her fear was even greater recently after some other kids started a fire near their house.

When she and her family went to a shopping mall, Jillian stayed close to her parents so that no one could snatch her. She was concerned when her mother went out that she might get lost.

Jillian was nearly hysterical as a little girl. She still woke up between midnight and two in the morning and did not feel safe. On those nights when her parents would not let her sleep on the floor of their room, she could not sleep all night. Jillian had to be careful about reading mystery books because they made her feel tense.

A whiz at learning, Jillian was a very fast reader with an excellent memory. Her mood was upbeat. She was always happy-go-lucky except when she was afraid at night. Jillian was helpful and very talkative. Like her sister Hayley and her father, she was also bursting with questions. She became very frustrated if she was unable to get out what she wanted to say. If she had something to say and others did not want to listen, she would yell it out anyway. "I have to let it out before I can relax."

She learned best when she did so through talking. It was a challenge for her to learn when not to talk, especially when she was excited about something. At those times she would want to tell her whole story in detail and other family members would be anxious for her to get to the point. Jillian did not handle teasing well. She enjoyed being active, playing soccer, dancing, and crocheting. Jillian had few physical problems except for hangnails and a wart on her foot.

We considered Jillian's fears to be her most outstanding feature. It is very unusual, in our experience, for a child to be so afraid that she could not even go to sleep at night. As with Hayley, we did not find the best medicine for Jillian the first time. We tried *Arsenicum album*, the medicine that helped Annie, as well as *Calcarea carbonica* (Calcium carbonate), another medicine for people who are preoccupied with safety issues. Neither of these two medicines had the profound effect on Jillian's fears that we had hoped.

Then, based specifically on Jillian's extraordinary fear of their house catching fire, undoubtedly her most unusual symptom, we gave her *Cuprum aceticum* (copper acetate). As with Hayley, the beneficial effects of Jillian's medicine lasted for a year, until she ate the same espresso-flavored cake. Jillian's mother called to report that the second dose of *Cuprum aceticum* worked the same day it was given. Once again Jillian's fear of fire diminished and she was able to sleep soundly.

River's Fears Started After He Watched a Ghost Story on TV

Ever since watching a scary ghost story on television five months earlier, five-year-old River was terribly fearful at night. It became a source of exhaustion for his mother. He hugged his blankets and stuffed animals. River began to complain of frightening dreams about monsters and bad wizards. His fear became so intense that he would not even go in his room alone during the day for fear that a monster would reach out from under the bed and grab him. When he woke with the nightmares, River could not fall asleep again unless his mother was by his side.

Homeopathy had helped River before with his recurring sinusitis and ear infections. Now his only real complaint, according to his mother, was his fearfulness. We prescribed *Stramonium* (thorn apple) for River. This is one of the excellent homeopathic medicines for frightened, clingy children. Their fears can often be traced to a particularly terrifying event such as the ghost show in River's case. We have seen a number of children with persistent fears after watching scary television programs, movies, or videos, and we encourage parents to be wary, especially with highly sensitive or impressionable youngsters.

River's mother called six weeks later to say that the *Stramonium* worked very well. River now went to his bedroom and the bathroom, even at night, without question. He was no longer waking up during the night and wanting his mother to put him back to sleep. His scary dreams disappeared and his life returned to normal.

27

―――⟨∞⟩―――

"She Climbs All Over Men"
Hypersexual Behavior

How can a parent tell what is normal sexual behavior for his or her child? The entire climate for youngsters has radically changed over the past generation. Sexual intercourse is common among many teenagers, epitomized by the debate about condoms in the schools. When is it appropriate and healthy for an individual to become sexually active? Human beings are capable of a broad range of sexual behaviors. What is considered normal or abnormal depends, to a large degree, on the prevailing cultural attitudes and societal values.[8]

The media introduces sex to our children at a very tender age. Some parents combat this tendency by eliminating television from their homes. AIDS is a very real threat to the lives of sexually active or drug-using adults and teenagers alike. A growing number of parents, appalled by how quickly children are being forced to grow up sexually and otherwise, are choosing to home-school their children to create a safer, more controlled learning environment. But how much can parents isolate their children from the currents of contemporary life?

---

[8] Schroeder, op. cit., 238.

Sexual abuse is another factor that directly affects the sexuality of youngsters. Shocking though the facts may be, many investigators agree that the prevalence of sexual abuse is approximately 25 percent of girls and 10 percent of boys.[9] This incidence increases with age. Among children who were sexually abused, 25 percent were under six years old, 34.3 percent ages six to eleven, and 40.6 percent ages twelve to seventeen. Sexually abused children often have a greater tendency to excessive masturbation and promiscuity. The long-term effects of sexual abuse can be devastating, including depression, self-destructive behavior, social isolation, eating disorders, anxiety, poor self-esteem, substance abuse, a tendency toward revictimization, relationship problems, and sexual dysfunction.[10]

As homeopaths, we find that there is a range of normal sexual behavior. The children in this chapter are excessively focused on sex. Children may grow out of this tendency or they may turn into sexually obsessed adults. Youngsters such as Chris, whose story follows, are more likely to be victims of sexual abuse whereas other children, especially those with both hypersexual and violent tendencies, may carry out sexual crimes. Or such children may simply place an overemphasis on sexual satisfaction in their intimate relationships.

Children exhibit excessive sexual behavior for many reasons. It is a mistake to assume the child has been sexually abused only because of frequent masturbation or sexual acting out. It is very important that parents communicate closely with their children in such cases in order to try to understand their personal issues as deeply as possible. If sexual abuse has indeed occurred, it is essential to seek immediate counseling for the family.

---

[9] Ibid., 242.
[10] Ibid., 245

With homeopathic treatment, as you can see in the following cases, the sexual sphere tends to shift into a more normal range as the whole child is brought into balance. The correct homeopathic prescription may save the individual from years of psychological pain and sexual dysfunction.

"Am I a Boy or a Girl?"

Chris was nine years old, blond, cute, and very inquisitive when he first came to see us. He was referred by a social worker because of his excessive masturbation. His birth parents had IQs of sixty-eight and seventy. His mother was obese and had worked as a stripper since she was seventeen. Chris' mother had no clear boundaries with him. She would kiss and fondle him inappropriately. When he was four, his mother complained that Chris masturbated excessively in public and was obsessed with touching his penis. The mother was accused of molesting Chris and he was sent to foster care. He told his foster mother he thought he was a girl. He played with Barbie dolls and dressed up his stuffed animals and put them to bed at night.

When we first saw Chris, he was in the fourth grade, but read at a first grade level. He had the comprehension of a five year old. He was unable to answer how long he had lived in his foster home, although he had been there for nine months. He had just been diagnosed with an undefined, extensive learning disability.

Chris seemed to masturbate all the time. He grabbed and pulled at his genitals no matter where he was. He left his clothes on and never exposed himself. Chris reacted very impulsively and lacked judgment. When his foster mother bought him a tool kit, he sawed off her front porch. When we asked Chris what he wanted to do when he grew up, he replied, "Grow up, get married, take off all my clothes, and have sex." He was simple-minded, but likable. Chris could understand "See the cat? See the dog?" but became lost when he read "See the dog chase the cat." He was still reading the third page of a book he began reading eight months before.

Chris was severely allergic to red food dye, which would cause him to vomit for three days. He slept like a rock and liked all kinds of foods.

We gave Chris a dose of *Bufo*. This toad is notorious, especially in Australia, for its hypersexual and inde-structible nature. These frogs reproduce so quickly that they are all over the Australian roads and, even when a driver accidentally runs over one with his car, they are not killed. *Bufo* is known to be an excellent homeopathic medicine for people who masturbate excessively and who have limited or delayed comprehension and learn-ing abilities, as seen earlier with Todd.

When Chris' foster mother brought him to see us one month later, she told us he was so normal that she couldn't remember why she brought him the first time. Before he could not read. Now he was up to second grade level, steadily improving, and had started to write in cursive. As far as she knew he had not masturbated at all since one week after taking the *Bufo*. He was no longer sensitive to red dye, and no longer darted out dan-gerously in traffic like before. His foster mother was even planning to get him a skateboard for his birthday. Though still in a developmentally delayed classroom, the teachers reported that he was much more normal and age appropriate. They were now optimistic about his catching up with the other children in intelligence and academic skills. Four months after taking the homeopathic medicine, Chris' report card said that he only needed to improve on his fractions. He was now up to fourth grade level. Everyone who knew Chris considered his improvement incredible. A report two years later found Chris in a permanent adoptive home and a regular classroom.

A Seductive Seven Year Old

Sally came into our office carrying her stuffed bunny. Her lips were painted red. Her mother, also a patient of ours for some time, brought Sally to us because the child kept touching her vagina. She told her mother it felt good. For over six months, she had walked around with her hand in her crotch. Whenever men came to their house, Sally hugged them, climbed all over them, and did not want to let go. She did this only with male visitors. She acted very manipulatively to get their attention. Sally's mother had a home sales business, and it was very embarrassing to her when Sally pounced on her customers. She masturbated frequently in the bathtub. She tried to lie on top of her girlfriend. She and her friend pretended they were having sex with animals.

Sally got along well with other children. She was quite boastful. She bragged to her friends, "I'm the only person who can swim in my friend's swimming pool" and "I have $125 in the bank." She wanted to impress. She also talked about wanting to have a lot of money and nice things when she grew up.

Sally had suffered from a number of episodes of strep throat and ear infections. She also complained of periodic headaches, which felt like a band around her forehead, and was bothered by abdominal pain while in the bathtub. Sally loved salt. She used to pour it into her hand and eat it plain.

We gave Sally *Platina,* made from platinum. People who need this medicine think, like the substance they need, that they are of great value and importance. They like to shine brightly and stand out above others. Their egotism can be excessive to the point of haughtiness. They may think they are more beautiful or better or even bigger than other people, as if they were of royal lineage. They may brag about wealth and fame, as Sally did with her friends. They have highly sexual natures and are often quite seductive. They sometimes complain of pains which feel like a band, just like Sally's headache.

When Sally returned to see us seven weeks later, her abdominal pain was gone. Her behavior around men was much improved. Sally told us, "I don't need to

Platina (platinum)

Children needing this medicine feel that, like platinum, their value is much greater than those around them. These children are boastful, particularly about money, and may pretend to have expensive things when they do not. They behave like royalty and tend to treat others as their slaves. Children matching the *Platina* state often exhibit seductiveness and sexual behavior beyond their tender years. As little girls, they often like to play dress-up and may dress provocatively. There is a precocious interest in the opposite sex. Numbness or voluptuous itching of the genitals may lead to early masturbation. Another common physical symptom is a bandlike sensation around the head or elsewhere.

climb all over them anymore because they're married." Not only did the *Platina* help Sally get over her inappropriate seductiveness, but she also became more self-confident and, according to her mother, "showed more real understanding and compassion for people who were hurting." She became better able to channel her energy into creative outlets and seemed happier in general.

The Little Boy Who Mooned

Austin's mother brought him to see us when he was five because she was worried about his sexually inappropriate behavior and his jealousy toward his baby sister. He had begun recently to use "bathroom language" to get attention. Austin had always been somewhat jealous of his younger sister. When their mother nursed her, Austin would hit the baby and put pillows over her head. He even pushed his sister down a flight of stairs once. He seemed to get a lot of satisfaction out of making his little sister cry. Austin was a "me first" kind of kid. He wanted to be served first and to get the biggest portion.

Most troubling to Austin's mother was his recent habit of mooning, both at home and in the school bathroom. He would pull his pants down in front of others and giggle without the slightest embarrassment. He played with his penis more than his mother considered to be normal and wanted to take off his clothes when a neighbor boy came over to play.

Austin loved to act silly and tell jokes. In the classroom, he acted like a clown and got into trouble repeatedly for teasing other children. He hummed and sang odd little songs that he made up. Austin's only physical symptom was a recurrent cough which happened every winter and lasted for six weeks.

Promiscuity is what stood out the most about Austin. Second in importance was his foolishness and silliness. We treated him with *Hyoscyamus* (Henbane), a medicine prominent for both of these symptoms. This is a medicine for people who act childishly and foolishly. They love to tease and attract attention. They may behave in a sexually teasing, but not really seductive, manner. It is one of the main homeopathic medicines for extreme jealousy after the birth of a sibling.

Austin's mother brought him back to see us two months later. Her report was quite positive. The bathroom talk was now infrequent. He no longer mooned. He had stopped playing excessively with his penis. He still wanted the most, but he was getting along better with his sister and had not acted violently toward her. Austin has not had a recurrence of his winter cough. He needed only one repetition of the *Hyoscyamus* nine months later and has done well since.

Hyoscyamus (henbane)

Children who need *Hyoscyamus* act excessively silly, joke, show off, talk too much, swear, and throw tantrums. They try to attract attention by whatever means available. Jealousy is a problem, especially when the younger brother or sister is born. The jealousy can lead to malicious violence against the younger child. These children are precocious sexually and may like to masturbate in public, run around naked, or expose themselves. Bedwetting may be a persistent complaint.

28

---- ⚭ ----

Most Commonly Asked Questions About Homeopathic Treatment

Many of these questions are answered in the text of the book. We have compiled them in one place here for your convenience.

➤ *Can homeopathy help me or my child with ADD?*

Most children with ADD can potentially benefit from homeopathic treatment; however, each case is individual. The cases in this book cover a wide range of behaviors and problems and provide a good idea of the scope of homeopathic practice. If you have reservations, specific questions, or your or your child's case is very complicated, call the homeopath first to make sure he or she feels that there is a good chance of homeopathy benefiting you.

➤ *My child's psychiatrist says his ADD is caused by a biochemical imbalance. Can homeopathy help him?*

Homeopathy believes that any biochemical imbalance is a result of an overall imbalance in a person rather than the cause of ADD. It is through bringing the whole person into balance that not only can the symptoms of ADD be improved, but most of the individual's other complaints as well. The goal of homeopathy is to bring deep and long-lasting balance into the person's life and health rather than just to regulate serotonin, dopamine, or some other neurotransmitter or chemical. When the person becomes balanced, the body's chemistry will automatically normalize as part of the overall healing process.

➤ *How long will I have to continue homeopathic treatment?*

Most patients need to continue under the care of a homeopath for at least two years. Significant progress is often noted within the first one to three months, as is evident in many of the cases that we have presented. Many people who are pleased with the results of their homeopathic treatment choose to use homeopathy for the rest of their lives.

➤ *How often will I need to see my homeopath?*

When first starting homeopathic treatment, visits are usually scheduled every five to eight weeks. After you or your child has responded well to treatment, your homeopath may only need to see you or your child two to three times a year to help you stay as healthy as possible and prevent future illness.

➤ *How often will the homeopathic medicine be given?*

Homeopathic medicines may be given in single doses, in which case the medicine will only be repeated or changed when symptoms arise. As long as you are responding well to the medicine you have been given, your homeopath will wait and let the healing process that has already begun continue to proceed. The medicines are also commonly prescribed on a daily or weekly basis. If you have been given a daily dose of homeopathic medicine, your homeopath may ask you to continue taking the medicine for weeks or months.

➤ *What is the difference between taking a single homeopathic medicine and the combination homeopathic medicines that I have seen in my health food store?*

There is only one homeopathic medicine at any point in time that will have the most dramatic effect on your healing. A trained and experienced homeopathic practitioner seeks to find that one specific medicine that most closely matches your symptoms. This exact or close match can produce profound and lasting healing. Combination medicines contain a variety of common homeopathic substances that have been found useful for such conditions as colds, flus, and sore throats. If the one medicine that you need is contained in that combination, you will respond well. If not, you will have no response or a partial response to the medicine.

Combination medicines should only be used for acute conditions when no qualified homeopath is available but should never be used for chronic or recurring conditions such as ADD and the other conditions mentioned in this book. The same is true of chronic physical ailments such as asthma, headaches, eczema, and arthritis. For such conditions, find a trained homeopath and you will be much more likely to be relieved of your suffering.

➤ *Are there side effects from homeopathic medicines?*

Homeopathic medicines are safe and gentle yet can produce powerful changes in people. There are no lists of side effects from particular homeopathic substances such as those from conventional medicines listed in the

Physician's Desk Reference (PDR). There are certain symptoms that a person may experience as part of his or her healing process. These include an aggravation (brief flare-up of already existing symptoms within the first week of taking a homeopathic medicine) and a return of old symptoms (brief re-experiencing of symptoms that you have had in the past). Both an aggravation and a return of old symptoms are usually an indication that the medicine is a good match for you and will be generally followed by a significant improvement in your chief complaint and overall state of health. On rare occasions an individual may experience a new symptom after taking a homeopathic medicine. If this happens, call your homeopath.

➤ *Can I begin homeopathic treatment while I am still taking conventional medication?*

The answer is generally yes, but this should be discussed with both your homeopathic practitioner and your prescribing physician.

➤ *How long do I need to avoid the substances and influences that interfere with homeopathic treatment?*

It is important to avoid these influences as long as you are being treated homeopathically. There have been reports of symptoms returning after exposure to such influences up to two years after taking the homeopathic medicine. If you have been helped significantly by homeopathy, it is probably best to play it safe and continue to avoid such exposure.

➤ *What if my child or I have food or environmental allergies?*

Homeopathy treats the whole person. When you are given a homeopathic medicine that closely matches your symptoms and state, you will experience greater energy and vitality and your immune system will become stronger. It is typical for patients who respond well to homeopathy to be able to go back to eating or being exposed to substances that bothered them prior to homeopathic treatment.

➤ *I can't get my son to stop eating junk food. Will homeopathy still work for him?*

Although it is much healthier for children to eat fresh, whole foods and to avoid the empty calories found in high sugar, fat, and processed foods, the right homeopathic medicine will still be effective for junk-food addicts.

➤ *Your cases sound extreme. Can homeopathy work for more "normal" children?*

Homeopathy can be beneficial to many people. Those with very extreme, intense symptoms tend to need medicines made from more intense substances in nature, such as rattlesnake, scorpion, rabies, and tarantula. Other milder, more even-tempered people may need more gentle medicines such as those made from flowers.

➤ *How can I find a qualified homeopath in my area?*

See "Referral Sources for Homeopathic Practitioners" in the Appendix.

➤ *What if there is no experienced homeopath in my area?*

Some homeopaths, such as ourselves, are very willing to treat patients by phone. They do so through exactly the same interview process as if you were to visit them in their offices. We have found the results are generally just as good as conducting the interview in person.

➤ *How do I know if my local homeopath practices the same way you describe in your book?*

Ask the practitioner if she practices classical homeopathy, uses one medicine at a time and spends at least one hour with the patient during the initial interview. The answer to all of these questions should be yes. Ask where the practitioner was trained. It should be an extensive course of at least 200 hours, and, preferably, two years or more, in addition to ongoing seminars, conferences, and training. Find out how long the person has been practicing homeopathy and what percentage of his or her practice is homeopathy. Look for a homeopath who graduated from an accredited or well-respected program of training and who devotes a minimum of 50 percent of her practice to homeopathy. Make sure that the practitioner is selecting medicines through an in-depth interview process rather than using machines, pendulums, or muscle testing to choose the medicine.

➤ *Can homeopathic medicines made from toxic substances ever poison the people taking them?*

Never. Homeopathic medicines are diluted one part to nine or ninety-nine parts from six to one hundred thousand times. The medicines carry the pattern of the original substance but, if tested, would never contain enough of the substance to be toxic or dangerous. Arsenic, snake venom, strychnine, and rabies are all homeopathic medicines, but are absolutely nontoxic as homeopathic medicines.

➤ *How expensive is homeopathic treatment?*

The only significant expense for homeopathic treatment is the office visits, which last from one to one and a half hours for the initial visit and approximately thirty minutes for follow-up visits. Cost depends on the experience and licensure of the practitioner. The cost of the homeopathic medicine itself is negligible. A year's worth of homeopathic medicine usually costs less than one prescription of many conventional medicines.

➤ *Are there insurance companies that cover homeopathic medicine?*

There are a few and the number is growing. As the public increasingly demands homeopathic care and insurance companies learn that homeopathic patients generally remain healthier and are much less costly to their insurance carriers, more providers will cover homeopathy. If your insurance provider does not cover homeopathic medicine, let the company know that you want coverage for homeopathic care or find another provider.

29

A Vision of Health and Balance for the 21st Century

We believe that by the year 2000 our society can find a far better way to treat ADD than drugging eight million children with stimulant medication. Many years ago we worked intensively with psychiatric patients and developmentally disabled children. It was our conviction then that there must be a better alternative than major tranquilizers to help these people to heal at a deep level. That is what led us to become naturopathic and homeopathic physicians. We still hold that conviction even more firmly and believe that homeopathy, along with other humane, natural therapies, may provide the answers to mental, physical, and emotional healing for many people.

Homeopathy works, plain and simple, and is very effective for many people with ADD and the other conditions included in this book as well as for most other health problems. In order to become acceptable to mainstream medicine, much more research is needed to provide concrete evidence regarding the effectiveness of homeopathic treatment of ADD. Funding for such research projects has not been available but will hopefully become a reality in the near future. We recently received a grant from the Homeopathic Community Council to compile a study of our best cases of ADD. Upon completion of the project, we hope, with the help of Jennifer Jacobs, MD, MPH, a pioneer in the field of homeopathic research, to apply for a grant to undertake a prospective study on the efficacy of homeopathic medicine to treat ADD.

In the meantime, practitioners such as ourselves choose to focus our attention on continuing to gather a wealth of clinical experience. We hope this book will enlighten healthcare professionals, patients, educators, parents, and others about the tremendous benefits of homeopathy. This safe, effective, natural, deep-acting, long-lasting, and cost-effective method of healing has the potential to benefit many millions of people, including those with ADD. We envision homeopathy as the medicine of the future.

—⌒⊗⊘⌒—

Appendix: Learning More

Recommended Books

ADD

Barkley, Russell, Ph.D. *Attention Deficit Hyperactivity Disorder: A Handbook for Diagnosis and Treatment.* New York: Guilford, 1990.

Greenhill, Lawrence L., and Betty B. Osman, Ph.D. (Eds.). *Ritalin: Theory and Patient Management.* New York: Mary Ann Liebart, 1991.

Hallowell, Edward M., M.D., and John J. Ratey, M.D. *Driven to Distraction.* New York: Simon and Schuster, 1994.

——— *Answers to Distraction.* : Pantheon, 1995.

Hartmann, Thom. *ADD Success Stories:* Grass Valley: Underwood Books, 1995.

——— *Attention Deficit Disorder: A Different Perspective.* Novato: Underwood-Miller, 1993.

Kelley, Kate, and Peggy Ramundo *You Mean I'm Not Lazy, Stupid or Crazy?!.* Cincinnati: Tyrell and Jerem, 1993.

Wender, Paul H., M.D. *Attention Deficit Hyperactivity Disorder in Adults.* New York: Oxford University, 1995.

———*The Hyperactive Child, Adolescent and Adult.* New York: Oxford University, 1987.

Homeopathy

Bellavite, Paolo and Signorini, Andrea. *Homeopathy: A Frontier in Medical Science.* Berkeley: North Atlantic, 1995.

Castro, Miranda. *The Complete Homeopathy Handbook.* New York: St. Martin's Press, 1990.

Ullman, Dana. *The Consumer's Guide to Homeopathic Medicine.* New York: Tarcher/Putnam, 1995.

——— *Discovering Homeopathy: Your Introduction to the Art and Science of Homeopathic Medicine.* Berkeley: North Atlantic, 1988, rev. 1991.

Ullman, Robert, and Judyth Reichenberg-Ullman. *The Patient's Guide to Homeopathic Medicine.* Edmonds, WA: Picnic Point Press, 1995.

Newsletters

The ADDed Line
3790 Loch Highland Pkwy.
Roswell, GA 30075
(800) 982-4028

Newsletter edited and published by Thom Hartmann, author of *ADD Success Stories* and *ADD: A Different Perspective.*

ADDult News
2620 Ivy Place
Toledo, OH 43613

Newsletter for adults with ADD.

Latitudes
1120 Royal Palm Beach Blvd. #283
Royal Palm Beach, FL 33411
(407) 798-0472

Bi-monthly newsletter of the Alternative Therapy Network devoted to alternative therapies for ADD, Tourette's syndrome, and autism.

Internet Homeopathic Resources

Website of Judyth Reichenberg-Ullman, N.D. and Robert Ullman, N.D.
http://www.healthy.net/jrru

Includes over 100 articles by the authors on homeopathy and holistic healing, audiotapes on treating various acute and chronic conditions with homeopathy, excerpts from *The Patient's Guide to Homeopathic Medicine* and *Ritalin-Free Kids: Safe and Effective Homeopathic Medicine for ADD and Other Behavioral and Learning Problems*, and the authors' conference and lecture schedule.

Health World on Line
http://www.healthy.net

Comprehensive on-line service specializing in information about alternative medicine. Includes journal articles, book excerpts, audiotapes, and on-line bookstore.

Homeopathy Home Page
http://www.dungeon.com/~cam/homeo/html
Includes many homeopathic worldwide homeopathic resources.

The ADD Forum on Compuserve
(Online, GO ADD)
Compuserve Information Service
(800) 524-3388, Representative 464

Provides discussion groups, conferences, and resource information 24 hours a day and includes over 45,000 members in more than 30 nations.

Homeopathic Book Distributors

The Minimum Price
250 H Street, P.O. Box 2187
Blaine, WA 98231
(800) 663-8272

Homeopathic Educational Services
2124 Kittredge Street, #71-Q
Berkeley, CA 94704
(510) 649-0294
(800) 359-9051 (orders only)

Referral Sources for Homeopathic Practitioners

International Foundation for Homeopathy (IFH)
P.O. Box 7
Edmonds, WA 98020
Tel: (206) 776-4147
Fax: (206) 776-1499
Directory of practitioners who graduated from the IFH Professional course.
Magazine, training programs, and annual case conference.

Homeopathic Academy of Naturopathic Physicians (HANP)
P.O. Box 69565
Portland, OR 97201
Tel: (503) 795-0579
Directory of naturopathic physicians board certified in homeopathy.
Journal and annual case conference.

The National Center for Homeopathy (NCH)
801 N. Fairfax, #306
Alexandria, VA 22314
Tel: (703) 548-7790
Fax: (703) 548-7792
Directory of licensed practitioners and study groups.
Magazine, training programs, annual conference, study groups, and general information about homeopathy.

Council for Homeopathic Certification (CHC)
1709 Seabright Avenue
Santa Cruz, CA 95062
(408) 421-0565
Directory of practitioners who have passed CHC certification examination.

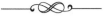

Glossary

acute illness—a condition that is self-limiting and short-lived, generally only lasting a few days to a couple of months.

aggravation—a temporary worsening of already existing symptoms after taking a homeopathic medicine.

alternative medicine—natural approaches to healing that are nontoxic and safe, including homeopathy, naturopathic medicine, chiropractic, acupuncture, botanical medicine, and many other methods of healing.

amphetamine—a substance, whether prescription or recreational, that stimulates the nervous system; includes Ritalin, Cylert, Dexedrine, diet pills.

antidepressant—a substance that alleviates depression.

antidote—a substance or influence that interferes with homeopathic treatment.

attention deficit disorder (ADD)—a diagnosis based on a constellation of symptoms that includes hyperactivity, attention problems, and/or impulsivity.

attention deficit hyperactivity disorder (ADHD)—synonymous with ADD.

auditory integration—a method of integrating brain function and hearing that originated in France.

autism—a diagnostic category that includes withdrawal, introversion, difficulty with social interaction, ritualistic behaviors, and limited verbal communication.

case taking—the process of the in-depth homeopathic interview.

C.H.A.D.D.—Children and Adults with ADD support group.

chief complaint—the main problem that causes a patient to visit a healthcare practitioner.

classical homeopathy—a method of homeopathic prescribing in which only one medicine is given at a time based on the totality of the patient's symptoms.

combination medicine—a mixture containing more than one homeopathic medicine.

constitutional treatment—homeopathic treatment based on the whole person, involving an extensive interview and careful follow-up.

conventional medicine—mainstream Western medicine that follows orthodox views of diagnosis and treatment.

Cylert—a stimulant medication used for children with ADD.

defense mechanism—that aspect of the vital force whose purpose is to maintain health and defend the body against disease.

developmental disability—mental or physical delays in development and maturity due to genetic or congenital abnormalities; previously called mental retardation.

Dexedrine—a stimulant medication used for children with ADD.

DSM-IV—published by the American Psychological Association, the diagnostic and statistical manual that classifies mental and emotional disorders into diagnostic categories.

Feingold diet—a dietary approach to treating ADD which includes the elimination of food colorings, additives, preservatives, flavorings, and salicylates.

gifted children—children classified with above-normal intelligence and learning abilities.

high potency remedies—remedies of a 200C potency or higher.

homeopathic medicine—a medicine that acts according to the principles of homeopathy.

homeopathic practitioner—an individual who treats people with homeopathic medicines according to the philosophy of homeopathy.

homeopathy—the use of a substance that causes a particular set of symptoms in a healthy person to relieve similar symptoms in a person who is ill.

Law of Similars—the concept that like cures like.

low potency remedies—remedies of a 30C potency or lower.

materia medica—a book that includes individual homeopathic remedies and their indications.

miasm—an inherited or acquired layer of predisposition.

minimal dose—the least quantity of a medicine that produces a change in the patient.

modality—those factors that make a particular symptom better or worse.

naturopathic physician—a physician who has graduated from a four-year naturopathic medical school and who treats the whole person based on the principle of the healing power of nature.

neurotransmitter—a chemical substance, like serotonin or dopamine, that transmits nerve impulses in the brain and nervous system, affecting thinking, behavior, sensory, and motor function.

nosodes—homeopathic medicines made from the products of disease.

obsessive compulsive disorder—a diagnostic category that includes symptoms of obsessive thought patterns and ritualistic behaviors.

phobia—an unreasonable, disproportionate, persistent fear of a specific thing.

potency—the strength of a homeopathic medicine as determined by the number of serial dilutions and succussions.

potentization—the preparation of a homeopathic medicine through the process of serial dilution and succussion.

prover—a person who takes a specific homeopathic substance as part of a specially designed homeopathic experiment to test the action of medicines.

provings—the process of testing out homeopathic substances in a prescribed way in order to understand their potential curative action on patients.

relapse—the return of symptoms when a homeopathic medicine is no longer acting.

remedy—a homeopathic medicine prescribed according to the Law of Similars.

repertory—a book that lists symptoms and the medicines known to have produced such symptoms in healthy provers.

return of old symptoms—the re-experiencing of symptoms from the past, after taking a homeopathic medicine, as part of the healing process.

Ritalin—a stimulant medication commonly used for ADD.

S.A.D.—School Avoidance Disorder (in other books this is also used as an abbreviation for seasonal affective disorder).

school refusal behavior—the refusal on the part of a child to go to school, usually associated with some type of fear.

simillimum—the one medicine that most clearly matches the symptoms of the patient and that produces the greatest benefit.

single medicine—one single homeopathic medicine given at a time.

state—an individual's stance in life; how he or she approaches the world.

stimulant—a substance, prescription or recreational, which stimulates the nervous system.

succussion—the systematic and repeated shaking of a homeopathic medicine after each serial dilution.

symptom picture—a constellation of all of the mental, emotional, and physical symptoms that an individual patient experiences.

tic disorder—a symptom picture characterized by twitches, jerks, and other convulsive or uncontrollable behaviors.

totality—a comprehensive picture of the whole person: physical, mental, and emotional.

Tourette's syndrome—a specific type of tic disorder that includes jerking, throat clearing, swearing, and other uncontrollable nervous system behaviors.

vital force—the invisible energy present in all living things that creates harmony, balance, and health.

Index

About the Authors

Judyth Reichenberg-Ullman, N.D., DHANP, M.S.W. and Robert Ullman, N.D., DHANP are licensed naturopathic physicians and board certified diplomates of the Homeopathic Academy of Naturopathic Physicians. Dr. Reichenberg-Ullman received a doctorate in naturopathic medicine from Bastyr University in 1983 and a master's in Psychiatric Social Work from the University of Washington in 1976. Dr. Ullman completed graduate work in psychology at Bucknell College in 1975 and received his N.D. degree from the National College of Naturopathic Medicine in 1981.

They are President and Vice President of the International Foundation for Homeopathy (IFH), instructors in the IFH Professional Courses and past faculty members of Bastyr University. They teach, write, and lecture widely. The couple co-authored *The Patient's Guide to Homeopathic Medicine,* which is used by homeopathic practitioners throughout the United States. It is available at local bookstores, through Picnic Point Press, 131 3rd Ave., N., Suite B, Edmonds, WA, 98020, or by calling Picnic Point Press at 1-800-398-1151.

Drs. Reichenberg-Ullman and Ullman are co-founders of The Northwest Center for Homeopathic Medicine in Edmonds, Washington where they specialize in homeopathic family medicine. They treat patients by phone consultation when there is no qualified homeopathic practitioner nearby. For consultations, call (206) 774-5599. Their website on the Internet at http://www.healthy.net/jrru contains many articles, book excerpts, teaching and lecture schedule and audiotapes of homeopathic treatments for various health problems.

They reside with their two lovable golden retrievers in Edmonds, Washington, just north of Seattle, which overlooks beautiful Puget Sound and the Olympic Mountains.